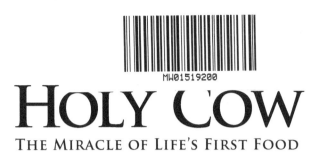

HOLY COW

THE MIRACLE OF LIFE'S FIRST FOOD

REDISCOVERING ANCIENT
IMMUNONUTRITION
FOR A MODERN WORLD

DOUGLAS A. WYATT

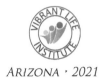

ARIZONA · 2021

Holy Cow: The Miracle of Life's First Food
Rediscovering Ancient Immunonutrition for a Modern World
by
Douglas A. Wyatt
Director of Research
Vibrant Life Institute

Published by
Vibrant Life Institute
a 501(3)(c) nonprofit organization

Printed in the United States of America

Vibrant Life Institute
2675 West SR89A #1095
Sedona, AZ 86336-5240
VibrantLifeInstitute.org
1st Edition, August 2021

Library of Congress Control Number: 2021902307

ISBN 978-1-736322-1-9

DISCLAIMER

This book is not intended as a substitute for the medical advice of physicians. The reader should regularly consult a physician in matters concerning his/her health, and particularly with respect to any symptoms that may require diagnosis or medical attention. The author and publisher are not responsible for any specific health or allergy needs that may require medical supervision or any damages or negative consequences arising from use of the treatments or ingredients described herein. Although the author and publisher have made every effort to ensure the information in this book is correct, the author and publisher disclaim any liability to any party for any loss or damages incurred as a result of reliance on said information.

The intention of this book is to tell the personal story of Kaye Wyatt's experience with bovine colostrum and to provide information for patients and their healthcare practitioners as they work hand-in-hand for optimal health outcomes. Neither the author nor the publisher assumes responsibility for any alleged loss or damage arising from any information, suggestions, or opinions expressed in this book.

Any specific references to products or companies are for historical reference only and should not be construed as endorsement or promotion of those products or companies by the author or publisher.

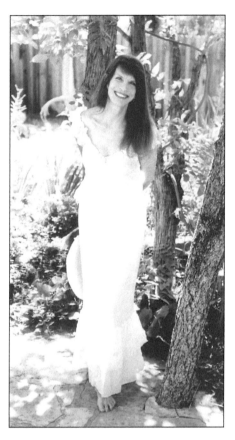

Kaye C. Wyatt

To Kaye:
Your life and our time together ended too soon, but I am
nonetheless grateful for both. Without you, there would
have been no re-discovery of bovine colostrum. You
gave life to the cause, and in doing so, you gave health
to millions of people around the world.

———◆———

To Mei Wei and Karen:
You are truly the force behind the scenes.

And to those seeking knowledge, hope, and healing:
May these pages shorten your journey to a healthier
state of being.

TABLE OF CONTENTS

He who has health has hope; and he who has hope
has everything.

Arabian Proverb

Why I Wrote This Book

Simply put, I want to create a movement that fundamentally changes the way medicine is taught and practiced in America. Quite a lofty goal for someone who is not a physician, but I think (and hope) that just might be my saving grace. I've been on this mission of sorts for quite some time, having been ignored or shut down over the years by people with lots of initials behind their names. As I look back on my seven decades with the present coronavirus pandemic staring us all in the face, I realize now is the time...Time to transform the present norm into a future filled with better patient outcomes, less physical and mental suffering, and vastly more vitality and resiliency.

Albert Einstein defined insanity as doing the same thing over and over again and expecting different results. We need to ask ourselves if medical insanity has stymied our innate healing mechanism, the immune system. Medical education hasn't changed much in the last half century, just more drugs to prescribe – a pill for this and a pill for that. Granted, there are life-saving drugs that have their time and place. But overuse, misuse, and abuse just might cause the ultimate "side effect." It seems as if the pharmaceutical companies develop new drugs for conditions they've invented, then convince people that they have these conditions, and then instruct people to demand their doctors give them the new drugs. What we need is a return to basics and common sense, both of which I will advocate in this book.

How did we get where we are today – in this predicament of our own making? In the 1940s, Oxford scientists Howard Florey and Ernst Chain transformed Alexander Fleming's newly-invented penicillin into a medically useful drug which saved countless lives and eventually led to the development of a plethora of antibiotics. With the advent of these new wonder drugs, we simultaneously started down a path of reliance on man-made drugs rather than the nature-made "drugs" that had been utilized for more than 4,000 years of recorded history. It is the living, breathing pharmaceutical factory – the dairy cow – so revered in Ancient Egypt and India for its life-giving nutrition and health sustenance. This original antibacterial and antiviral powerhouse was abandoned by Western medicine in the mid-20th century and now calls us to renew and refocus our attention. It is often said that what is old and forgotten shall become new again, and so this is my story of rediscovery and renewal.

The first part of my life was influenced by my military service in Vietnam as a Marine Corps helicopter pilot followed by various jobs in the financial sector, including stock trader, real estate franchisee, and marketing consultant. At the time, none of this piqued my interest in health, but it did provide business acumen that would later prove valuable. My early health knowledge was limited to what I learned from my mother, an herbalist, and from spending summers on my grandfather's ranch in Idaho. Unbeknownst to me at the time, the life-affirming experience of calving on the ranch would later point me in the direction of my life's true mission.

After suffering most of her life from a failed immune system, Kaye Chytraus entered my life. If by chance or by fate, her unfortunate lack of health led to my good fortune of rediscovering an ancient health remedy – colostrum – a mother's first milk and the "gift of life." Kaye later became my wife and together we worked tirelessly to understand this amazing substance as it related to immune health. No one doubts the power of the human immune system, least of all me, but I experienced firsthand just how critical colostrum is to immune resiliency and the healing power that bovine colostrum offers.

This book is the story of my journey to help my ailing wife, her journey towards better health, and our shared vision of healing and resiliency for all those affected by physical or mental disease or the misguided treatment of said disease. Despite our many scientific and medical advances, people are sicker and suffering more today from autoimmune and inflammatory-related diseases. Stemming the epidemic of chronic disease is paramount, yet the emergence of SARS-CoV-2 reminds us of the lurking dangers of highly infectious pathogens. Immune resiliency is more important than ever before, and the good news is that colostrum has a significant role to play. It is often said that the simplest solution is the best solution. For all its simplicity, colostrum is our best solution.

I invite you to join me on this journey – the journey of rediscovery that reminds us how vital colostrum has been throughout human history and how it may hold the key to the survival of our species henceforward. I will make the case that bovine colostrum is the nutritional imperative for optimal health and immune resiliency in the face of ever-changing environmental threats and unknown immune challenges. If you are in the medical profession, I hope that the ideas I present will make you question some of what you've been taught and provide you with a new perspective on treating modern day ills. If you are a health consumer, I aim to teach you the importance of health sovereignty by which you will gain knowledge and inspiration to take charge of your own health and become the healthy, resilient person you are destined to be. Colostrum is the "gift of life" for newborns and the "gift of health" for adults I wish to share with you.

Learn to light a candle in the darkest moments of someone's life. Be the light that helps others see; it is what gives life its deepest significance.

Roy T. Bennett

INTRODUCTION
Is Anyone Listening?

Two and a half millennia ago, the Father of Medicine said, "All disease begins in the gut." I often wonder what Hippocrates' contemporaries thought of his bold declaration. Did they listen? Did it affect their understanding or practice of ancient medicine? And then I ask myself what happened between then and now – did we forget about Hippocrates, or worse, ignore him? Modern (Western) medicine's realization that there's a strong connection between gastrointestinal health and immune resiliency is rather recent, and not all medical practitioners have come around to this concept. Yet this appears to be the emerging future of modern medicine, especially if we expect to survive the next millennia.

According to the Centers for Disease Control and Prevention (CDC), six in ten American adults have a chronic disease and four in ten have two or more chronic diseases.[1] Most physicians agree that nearly every American will die of an autoimmune disease, whether heart disease, cancer, diabetes, lung disease, depression, or Alzheimer's disease. Wow! That's dismal. I would add that when death comes, it comes prematurely and with a whole lot of prolonged physical and mental pain, not to mention the family burden. So, if you are one of the millions suffering with some type of autoimmune or chronic disease, you should know up front, that I find this absolutely unacceptable. You should also know that I am quite passionate when it comes to health sovereignty – the power and responsibility that each of us possess over our own bodies and health destiny. Given the choice, no one says, "I'll take heart disease, a little asthma, and throw in type 2 diabetes for good measure." But this unfortunate reality contributes to decreased life expectancy and unnecessary suffering.

Unless we advocate dramatic changes in our approach to health and disease, we cannot move past being our own worst enemies. And so, the concept – or perhaps more of a mindset – of health sovereignty is something that I'll come back to time and time again throughout our journey together. You have just one physical body, and your one all-important task is to take as good care of it as you can – feed it well, exercise it regularly, and stimulate its mind. At your birth and throughout childhood, it was your parents' responsibility; but now that you've taken ownership, don't give up the responsibility nor the right to every organ, every tissue, and every cell it possesses.

This was true for my beloved Kaye. She was born in the 1940s, a time in which ionizing radiation (X-rays) as a medical treatment was in its prime, although it had been in use as early as the 1910s. Irradiation was particularly useful for getting human tissue to shrink (by literally killing cells), and it was thought that low-dose radiation was safe. Of course, it was later discovered to lead to cancer. Thousands of servicemen in World War II underwent irradiation therapy, and an estimated 500,000 to 2 million civilians were treated over nearly three decades beginning in the early 1940s, with the majority being children when they were first treated.[2] The medical profession utilized irradiation therapy for a host of childhood conditions, including an enlarged thymus gland, noisy breathing, wheezing in the chest, asthma, cough, runny nose, tonsillitis, ear infections, birth marks, moles, and acne.

During the first half of the twentieth century, there was a misconception among physicians that if an infant had an enlarged thymus gland, he or she had a high risk of suffocation and or sudden death (SIDS).[3] An enlarged thymus occurs naturally during an upper respiratory tract infection, and it also causes a sore throat. So, if an infant was prone to these infections, the family physician commonly irradiated it as a way to get the gland to shrink and relieve the child's excessive crying from the pain. This "therapy" is known as Nasopharyngeal Radium Irradiation (NRI).

Complicating the situation was mothers' complete trust in the physician (the "God complex"). What the physicians didn't know at the time was that during an upper respiratory tract infection, the thymus gland produces T-cells (immune cells) to help fight off the infection. This normal immune process causes the gland to swell up and appear enlarged. It was a case of this new therapy being the "truth" – an effective, and presumably life-saving medical treatment – at that moment in time. The 1940s and 1950s saw peak utilization of NRI before it was discontinued in the mid to late 1960s.

As an infant and young child, Kaye had numerous infections and believing that this may cause crib death, her family physician irradiated her thymus gland. As a result, Kaye's immune system was nearly wiped out. It could no longer fight infections on its own, and she was not alone. Of the thousands of infants and children irradiated, many lives were cut short or filled with immense pain and suffering; many later developed throat cancer. And it wasn't only the fate of the children, but many physicians died of radiation poisoning.

Going forward, Kaye's non-functioning immune system took a heavy toll. Every cold, every bug that came along weakened Kaye, and she would subsequently suffer with bouts of bronchitis and bacterial pneumonia. The vicious cycle continued as physicians gave her more and more powerful antibiotics to fight the infections, which in turn, destroyed much of the beneficial bacteria in her gut. It also put her on the path to leaky gut, something no one knew about at the time.

I likened her situation to being on permanent chemo-therapy. Kaye's body was dying a slow and painful death. Our desperation ran deep, as no herbal or homeopathic medicine, Chinese herbs, or acupuncture helped. By 1992, Kaye's immune system was in shambles; she was physically and mentally devastated. One day, Kaye asked me to help her die.

The immune system is like the software that runs the human body. From time to time, we may get a little bug (i.e., a virus that causes the common cold) that brings on the sniffles, a runny nose, or a sore throat. The software's "self-fix code" is activated and in a few days, we're feeling better and back to our normal routines. In a nutshell, that's immune resiliency. The immune system is very efficient, so most of the time, we don't give it a second thought…that is until something goes really wrong, as in the case of an immunodeficiency disorder.

An immunodeficiency disorder disrupts the body's natural ability to defend against pathogens, including viruses, bacteria, and parasites. Some people are born with immunodeficiency disorders, but far more are acquired later down the road. In Kaye's situation, it was as if her software and her gut microbiome were periodically getting attacked by malware – the antibiotics – that killed the good bacteria and made the bad bacteria stronger. At the time, very few people realized the significance of an unbalanced microbiome or even knew a gut microbiome existed.

When Hippocrates said that all disease begins in the gut, he just might have inferred that it's all the crap we put into our guts that compromises the immune system and causes disease. That crap includes antibiotics, the ones that are typically over-prescribed and the ones that are ubiquitous in our food supply – those that come from conventional farming when non-sick meat animals are fed or injected with antibiotics. Prescription and over-the-counter pain medications…more crap. Chemical pesticides, herbicides, and hundreds of environmental toxins…more crap. High-sugar foods, processed foods, fast foods…more crap. With about eighty percent of the immune system residing in the gut, all this malware overloads the immune system to the point at which resiliency can no longer be maintained.

And just like when your computer starts running a little slow or acting a little strange, you've got a gut feeling that something is wrong. But you limp along because you're either too busy to get it repaired or you don't want to spend the money to get it fixed, and then one day, it won't even power up. That's more or less what happens to your body after years of malware…a total shutdown and an "oh, shit" moment.

We may be broken and immunocompromised, but we don't have to be if we choose health sovereignty. If we reach for immune resiliency, we can achieve it…by taking bovine colostrum AND by removing the toxins from our internal and external environments AND by adopting healthy lifestyle behaviors. It's up to us to rid ourselves of the malware, install anti-virus software, get regular tune-ups, and we'll run smoothly and consistently for years to come.

Kaye's lack of health was a symptom of imbalance and immunodeficiency, and the radiation that had rendered her thymus gland non-functional was just one piece of the puzzle. The other was that her mother did not breastfeed her. While it is not my intention to chastise any woman who – for whatever reason – does not or cannot breastfeed her child, I will vigorously make the case for the importance of breastfeeding. As a society, we have a vested interest in whether our children receive colostrum and breastmilk, and I hope that by the time you reach the end of this book, you too will advocate for breastfeeding, whether you are a biological mother or father, or not.

All mammalian species are capable of breastfeeding their young and with the exception of humans, offspring will not survive without their mothers' colostrum and breastmilk. The passive immunity conveyed to newborn animals via colostrum is vital to their immediate survival. This is best illustrated by the wild gazelle born on the African savannah – the same savannah that is home to prey animals scouting their next meal. If a newly birthed gazelle is to have any hope of outrunning a hungry lioness, she must get up on all four legs with the steadiness and strength to keep up with the rest of the herd. She must also maintain calm and quiet so as not to attract the lioness with her bleating. Such is the function of a mother's colostrum. The bioactive components – which I'll discuss in greater detail later – are responsible for a wide range of functions critical to both surviving and thriving.

Not having received the myriad of breastfeeding benefits and having her thymus gland irradiated disadvantaged Kaye for much of her early life. Our rediscovery of colostrum helped restore her health and desire to continue living – something that I was profoundly thankful for at the time. I couldn't imagine my life without her, and the day she asked me to help her die…I would never wish such pain and agony on anyone. In retrospect, I realize that the two of us were on a spiritual journey of sorts – one in which God was playing a behind-the-scenes role that began by bringing the two of us together and nudging us in the right direction towards colostrum. Faith and prayer brought all this to fruition, and we felt so blessed that we wanted to share it with the world.

In his ancient wisdom, Hippocrates offers medical insight which remains profound today. "If someone wishes for good health, one must first ask oneself if he is ready to do away with the reasons for his illness. Only then is it possible to help him." So, I ask you: Are you immune-resilient or are you immunocompromised? Are you listening to what your gut is telling you? Are you ready to take this journey with me?

By living a life based on wisdom and truth,
one can discover the divinity of the soul,
its union to the universe, the supreme peace
and contentment which comes from satisfying the
inner drive for self discovery.

Ancient Egyptian Proverb

1

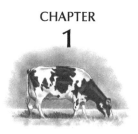

Living in Today's World
Requires a Strong Immune System

Immune resiliency is the most significant determinant of human survival. I believe it's the key health lesson from the COVID-19 pandemic and every pandemic past, present, and future. A robust and balanced immune system allows individuals to respond to pathogenic threats with an appropriate immune/inflammatory response without becoming so overwhelmed as to succumb to the cytokine storm. Pathogens have been a part of our environment since the dawn of time, and DNA from viruses is present in our own DNA. Viruses adapt, or die. We adapt, or die. And for the bacterial pathogens that we are able to eliminate, we should use the most precise technology available. There's no need for a machine gun when a rifle will do. It's really quite simple.

A million years of evolution has taught us the importance of passive immunity – immunity to pathogens created through the transfer of antibodies from another person or animal via the birth mother's colostrum and milk. Passive immunity is the reason all mammals, with the exception of humans, can exist at all. This astute conclusion is something my mentor, medical anthropologist John Heinerman, Ph.D. taught me. Rather than looking at colostrum as just a substance with a lot of wonderful "stuff" in it, Dr. Heinerman gave me a way to view colostrum through the eyes of a sociologist and an anthropologist with all the history of mankind and the origins of the very first mammals.[4]

Before I delve into the nitty-gritty of what is actually in colostrum, I need to explain what colostrum is. I've received many blank stares and silently nodding heads, and I've definitely made the assumption that colostrum is as well-known as say cholesterol, for example. Yet, there was a day some decades ago that the term *cholesterol* was not part of our vernacular. And while I was going on and on about how great colostrum is, some brave soul would shyly interrupt and ask, "*Is colostrum like cholesterol?*" Colostrum is too important to be confused with cholesterol, yet certainly less of a physician-patient discussion topic than one's cholesterol numbers. That is something I aim to change. By the time physicians finish reading this book, I hope they'll recommend colostrum to every patient in their practice, and the non-physicians will educate their family, friends, and personal physicians about colostrum.

Colostrum is a milk-like substance that is produced by the mammary glands of mammals just prior to and a few days after the birth of their newborn. Colostrum is known by many other names, including pre-milk, foremilk, first-milk, beestings, bisnings, and one I have particular affinity for – "first food of life." Mammalian mothers provide colostrum to their newborns as an initial source of food and of immune bioactives and growth factors, including antibodies and immunoglobulins which protect the infant from disease. Human colostrum is slightly yellowish in color, somewhat sticky in texture, and very concentrated. Because the newborn has a small stomach and immature digestive tract, a mother's colostrum is a low-volume secretion, unlike breast milk. In other words, a little goes a long way, which also means that every drop of colostrum is precious. Colostrum goes to work immediately by transferring immunity and initiating immune function followed by maturing the G.I. tract and sealing up the newborn's leaky gut. I've detailed this very important function in Chapter 2. Colostrum also has a mild laxative-like effect which helps stimulate the first stool (meconium) to be passed.

A mother produces colostrum for about three days, after which the colostrum begins to taper off and "true milk" replaces it. This is one reason why it's so vital to attempt breastfeeding early and repeatedly if necessary. All of the wonderful "stuff" in colostrum works synergistically to protect and prepare the infant for life outside the safe, secure, and sterile environment of its mother's womb. After about five or six days, colostrum production has completely ceased and is replaced by breast milk which continues to be produced by the mammary glands as long as the child suckles the breast. Because breast milk does contain some immune bioactives and growth factors, although significantly less than colostrum, extended breastfeeding provides on-going benefits for the infant.

Colostrum is very frequently assumed to be "milk" or in the case of bovine colostrum, a dairy product, and I've had many heated discussions about this. Colostrum is not milk! According to the U.S. Pasteurized Milk Ordinance, if animal milk contains colostrum, it is an "abnormality of milk" and deemed unsuitable for sale.[5] The California Food and Agricultural Code, section 35602 clarifies this further by defining cow and goat milk for human consumption as that which is collected on the sixth day after the calf's birth.[6] The U.S. government says that colostrum is something other than milk, and only the dairy farmers (not the milk producers) are able to collect colostrum, so why the misidentification? It probably has something to do with both colostrum and milk coming from the breast and all the colloquial terms we have for colostrum – pre-milk, fore-milk, and first-milk.

Colostrum is its own unique secretion expressed from the breast of female mammals. For more evolved mammalian species such as humans and other primates, I would add that – in the spiritual sense – colostrum is an expression of a mother's love for the child that she has carried for nine months and just brought into the world. Once we learn about what is in colostrum and how its synergistic bioactive components impart a strong foundation for one's future growth and immune health, we can't help but look upon colostrum as a mother's gift to her newborn child.

The biology of colostrum development within the mammary gland gives me pause when I think about how it comes to be. Colostrum is blood serum that is activated by the mammary cells; the mother's blood serum is rich in immunoglobulins which are some of the most significant immune-imparting substances in colostrum. Colostrum is expressed by mammary secretory cells and each "droplet" is encased in a tiny fat globule surrounded by a portion of the mammary cell membrane (*See Figure 1*).

During this process, each secretory cell produces colostrum globules by pinching off a piece of the cell membrane, and the components that the cell will use to produce colostrum are incorporated into small vesicles. These vesicles will be processed through the Golgi apparatus and the endoplasmic reticulum, two specialized organelles in the cell that are fueled by the mitochondria. The cell's nucleus contains the DNA which codes for all the proteins produced within the organelles. The end-product is the colostrum-fat globule which exits the cell and eventually travels to the milk duct in the breast. The membrane that surrounds the colostrum-fat globule helps protect the colostrum from the normal digestive action of the gastrointestinal tract; it allows the colostrum bioactives to reach the small intestine intact where they'll have the most significant health-enhancing impact. This protective membrane is important to colostrum's effectiveness and also a key player in the manufacturing of colostrum supplements. Keep this in the back of your mind because I'll return to it in Chapter 9.

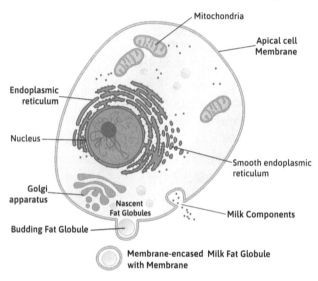

Figure 1: Mammary Secretory Cell

I didn't write this book for cellular biologists per say, so here's an easier way to understand the process of how colostrum and breast milk are made: Think of it like an automated bakery that is making a basic cake. The vesicle is the mixing bowl that holds the raw ingredients (components which will later become colostrum) and is brought into the kitchen along a conveyor belt; the Golgi apparatus is the mixer and the endoplasmic reticulum is the oven; the mitochondria is the natural gas that runs the entire bakery and the nucleus is the cookbook which holds the recipe (DNA) to make the cake. The colostrum-fat globule is the finished cake, and the outer membrane is the plastic wrap that encases the cake and keeps it fresh until you're ready to eat it.

As mentioned previously, passive immunity from mother to offspring is important in creating a strong immune system and immune resilience. In humans, some of this immunity comes from maternal antibodies which are transferred through the placenta to the fetus, and the rest is conveyed through colostrum and breast milk. In other mammalian species and specifically cows, for this discussion, all of the immunity is conveyed through colostrum. Unlike humans, cows do not have the ability to nurse their young longer than a few days, hence a higher concentration of antibodies transfers in a shorter period of time. In our bakery example, bovine colostrum is a four-layer cake, and human colostrum is a single-layer cake. Because bovine colostrum is like a "super-charged" immune concentrate that is biologically transferrable, humans and all other mammalian species, any immunocompromised – or healthy – human, primate, dog, cat, rabbit, etc. can utilize bovine colostrum as a nutritional supplement.

When I say that living in today's world requires a strong immune system, I don't think many people would disagree. They may disagree on how to achieve immune resilience and may even disagree on the importance of colostrum. While it is true that humans won't die if they don't receive their mother's colostrum – that's a good thing since not every newborn is breastfed – there's no valid reason to not advocate for breastfeeding. I speak about the benefits of colostrum as I witnessed first-hand with my beloved wife Kaye, and later, countless times with countless other people, many of whom shared their most personal stories of desperation and despair.

When Kaye told me that she was physically and

mentally exhausted from her repeated bouts with illness and she wanted to die, I was devastated. I was completely unprepared and emotionally impotent. Not even the horrors of Vietnam could compare to hearing her pleading words, *"Doug, I need you to help me die."* The only thing we had left was prayer, and so we turned to God in earnest. And God heard us.

I considered us quite blessed at the time because our prayers were answered the following day. I was meeting with a colleague who noticed that I wasn't really present… that although my body was sitting in front of him, my mind was somewhere else. He said, *"Doug, you're not here with me this morning. We're not going anyplace, and I want you to talk about it. I know that might be difficult, but something is really going on with you."* So, I began to tell him about Kaye, and almost immediately, he asked, *"Doug, have you heard about colostrum?"*

Colostrum? Colostrum? As my mind began racing, I realized what I already knew. Having spent summers on my grandfather's ranch, I remembered that from time to time, a calf would die from scours if it didn't receive its mother's colostrum within the first twenty-four hours of being born. Scours caused by bacterial or viral infections leads to extensive, life-threatening diarrhea in neonatal calves. Yet, calves who successfully nursed received the immune bioactives in colostrum that in turn, eliminated pathogens in the G.I. tract and established a robust foundation for the cow's immune system going forward in life. Colostrum conveyed immunity…could it really be that simple?

In that moment, it was like a bolt of lightning from the heavens. Upon reflection, it was a heaven-sent blessing. Colostrum was – and is – software for the immune system and for robust physical and neurological development. I'm grateful to my colleague for reminding me about the immune system being passed on from mother to baby. His background was in naturopathic medicine, and he had received extensive training in Belgium at a time when preventative and "alternative" medicine were more widely accepted there than in the United States. In fact, the extent of American alternative practitioners was pretty much confined to promoters of veganism and herbal remedies; bovine products would have been considered a sacrilege.

I felt further blessed when he told me that a local dairy farmer was giving him fresh colostrum, and he was drying it in his kitchen for personal use. So, I bought a quarter pound of the dried colostrum with the intention of surprising Kaye with my heaven-sent gift. My colleague also gave me a few scientific abstracts detailing colostrum's anti-inflammatory action, injury repair, pain relief, gastrointestinal benefits, and immune support. I took my gifts home to Kaye and was met with: "*You paid what… for what? You take it back!*" Needless to say, she wasn't as happy as I thought she would have been. I was disheartened, but had faith…and a little something up my sleeve. Instead of returning the colostrum, I hid it away, but I left the scientific abstracts strategically placed so Kaye would surely happen upon them. And then I waited. She did, and I didn't have to wait long.

A mere couple of days later while on a morning walk, Kaye sprained her knee so badly that she literally crawled back home. After a trip to the E.R. where she was given a wrap-on support to stabilize the swollen knee joint, she said in a moment of frustration, "*Okay, I'll take some of your dang stuff…your dang medicine.*" Kaye took a couple of teaspoons and went to bed in a lot of pain with her black and blue, swollen knee all wrapped up. I really hoped that she (and I) would get some much-needed sleep.

I was up early the next morning, drinking my coffee and reading the newspaper at the kitchen table, when Kaye walked in. "*Kaye!*" I exclaimed. Still half asleep, she answered, "*What?*" Again, I exclaimed, "*Kaye!*" and she retorted, "*What?*"

I pointed. *"Your leg."* As Kaye pulled up her nightgown and looked down at her knee, she uttered a bewildered, *"Huh?"* Not only had she removed the support sometime during the night, but the swelling was down, the discoloration was gone, and she wasn't feeling any pain. Neither of us could believe it. We sat together in amazement, relishing in the moment... wondering if we had just experienced a miracle.

But that wasn't the only miracle we would be given. Kaye continued taking the colostrum – certainly no reason to mess with a good thing, and we were eager to learn more. A few days later, Kaye's chronic, low-grade fever broke. This was the very same fever that had plagued her for the previous decade. As a result of her immunocompromised state, she couldn't rid her body of the constant infections, but this was the turning point. This amazing sequence of events was the answer to our prayers.

I can honestly say that colostrum effected the most profound change in Kaye's life... in our lives... and in my life. We now had hope for the future, and that heart-breaking request Kaye had made of me could be put out of our minds. The changes in Kaye's health were startling and being well more of the time than being sick was transformational for her as an individual. She no longer needed antibiotics every few months for the bouts of pneumonia that tagged along with every cold or flu virus. She made colostrum an integral part of her daily regimen, as if reading the morning paper, brushing her teeth, or snuggling with me on the couch. At the first inkling of a cold, she'd take a little extra colostrum and by the next morning, she'd feel one-hundred percent better – as if the virus was completely and miraculously repelled.

Anyone who has overcome a significant health challenge realizes just how wonderful life can be as they go forward. Unfortunately, there are a lot of unwell people as a consequence of being immunocompromised, which manifests in many forms and individualistic ways. They are your friends, neighbors, co-workers, children, parents, and complete strangers who don't know what to do or where to turn. It may even be YOU. Multiple doctors who can't pinpoint a medical problem; multiple conditions; vague symptoms; symptoms masked by certain medications; the treatment is as bad or worse than the condition; or the ultimate patient insult – a psychiatry referral from a frustrated doctor. But I want people to have hope that physical and mental suffering need not be ubiquitous, and there is a path forward. After the decades of disappointment and disability, Kaye was ready for a new adventure, as was I, and we embarked on an expedition to learn as much as we could about colostrum.

In the early days of the Internet (the "dark ages") and the time before PubMed, the only way of accessing medical literature was through the library of a local medical school. Fortunately, we lived in Salt Lake City near the University of Utah. The bad news was that not just anyone could gain access to the library; you had to be a student or a doctor and since Kaye and I were neither, we lamented but asked for divine help. What we received was nothing short of miraculous. I met a woman named Debbie who for a reason unbeknownst to me, decided to share her story with me.

"My husband has been home and in bed for three weeks. He's on enormous quantities of antihistamines, and every drug that the doctors can find. He has massive allergies. He has hives all over his body…down his esophagus, inside and out, clear throughout him. He can't even stand to have a sheet touch him, can't stand to have his clothes touch him, can't eat because his whole mouth and all his insides are full of hives, and they itch and they're painful and they're killing him. They're driving him crazy."

Debbie was obviously anguished and after hearing her story, I brought her home to Kaye. We gave Debbie some colostrum to try out on her husband. Neither of us was sure that it could help but the situation sounded so desperate, anything was worth a try. A day and a half later, we heard a knock at our door. Debbie was standing there with tears of joy running down her face – for she had her own miracle to share. Her husband's hives had all disappeared.

Mind you, I wasn't in the habit of bringing other women home with me, but this was a worthy and rewarding exception. Divine intervention struck again. Debbie was a medical researcher who had access to the University of Utah Medical School's library. She gave us a library card so we could access all the literature we could find on colostrum, much of which was related to animal husbandry in veterinary journals and the specific bioactive components identified in colostrum. Our search turned up thousands of peer-reviewed articles that had been published on various types of colostrum, particularly bovine and ovine (sheep). The sheer volume of clinical research and the information contained within was absolutely staggering to us. The information we compiled provided us with the foundation from which we could begin educating people about colostrum's beneficial effects on a wide range of conditions – well beyond the personal success we experienced with Kaye's immune system.

Kaye and I were the pioneers of colostrum and its "rediscovery," and together, we founded The Center for Nutritional Research, a not-for-profit organization dedicated to the continued research and promotion of bovine colostrum. But our journey was far from over. Colostrum wasn't something you could just go pick up at the local market. In fact, there were no sources of commercial colostrum anywhere in the United States which met the stringent standards set by the USDA for the handling of milk intended for human consumption. Colostrum was actually considered a waste product by most dairy farmers who would leave it in a can by the side of the road for animal feed companies to pick it up. The colostrum would be processed and dehydrated and resold back to dairy farmers who fed it to the next season's newborn calves when their mothers could not provide enough colostrum.

When I think back of how colostrum was considered "waste"– something to be discarded – I shudder. Dr. Heinerman taught me that colostrum (and mother's milk) held great prominence for early civilizations, and even documented in their ancient texts. Egyptian hieroglyphs depict Hathor, the cow goddess and symbol of rebirth, suckling the pharaoh. For Ancient Egyptians, colostrum was considered the *elixir of metamorphosis* which conferred immortality to the pharaoh. The Great Divine Mother Isis was also a cow goddess, and she is depicted as the mother and nurse of the pharoahs. Images of "Milk-Giving Isis" (*Isis Lactans*) are prevalent and depict the king suckling at the three most significant and symbolic times – birth (life), coronation (power, wisdom, and divinity), and rebirth (renewal).[7]

Interestingly, milk from the cow goddesses wasn't limited to just the pharoah's benefit. It was also used in Ancient Egyptian healing, and specifically the milk of a woman who birthed a son, as a medicinal ingredient. Milk was used for topical burns to "extinguish the fire." Hieroglyphs suggest that if you applied Isis' divine milk to a burn, she would heal you and the fire would leave your body. Today, soaking a burn in cool milk or applying a milk compress is a common home remedy for slight to moderate burns. Our modern understanding of colostrum and milk conveying immunity and facilitating healing suggests that the Egyptians were on to something, even if they didn't know exactly why. My journey with Kaye sought to answer those very questions about immunity and healing and whether it was possible to make colostrum available to people who needed some divine intervention.

2

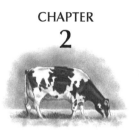

Milk is Good for Mammals

Child rearing practices change over time and subject to whomever is considered the "expert" or influencer of the day. In modern times, the length of breastfeeding has been determined by social norms, mothers returning to the workplace, and the successful marketing of infant formulas. From 1900 to 1960, negative attitudes caused a significant decline in breastfeeding, but the trend has been reversing in the U.S. according to CDC data.[8] In 2016, 83.8% of infants received some breastfeeding, up from 76.1% in 2009 and at twelve months of age, 36.2% were still receiving at least some breastmilk, compared to 24.6% seven years earlier. Even though breastfeeding trends are going in the right direction, just over 15% of children never receive the health benefits of their mothers' colostrum and milk, and this is cause for concern.

If you are a mom-to-be or you know someone who is, I urge you to take this chapter to heart as I make the case for early and extended breastfeeding. I also encourage you to consult with a certified birth doula and/or lactation specialist, as they provide breastfeeding guidance and support. La Leche League International (llli.org) is a good resource to learn more about breastfeeding benefits and various issues that arise for new mothers. Being well-informed at this special time can make childbirth a little easier, especially if it's a first child.

According to the American Academy of Pediatrics, infants should be exclusively breastfed for the first 6 months followed by continued breastfeeding plus age-appropriate complementary foods for one year or longer.[9] The World Health Organization has a similar recommendation but increases the length of continued breastfeeding up to two years of age or beyond.[10] I would add to these recommendations that a new mom initiate breastfeeding within an hour of giving birth so that her newborn receives colostrum at the earliest possible moment. Since colostrum is expressed in the first seventy-two hours, after which it tapers off, it's important for baby to receive the maximum quantity (and benefit). Every drop of mother's colostrum is as precious as her newborn.

The reason that colostrum is so important to a newborn lies in the fact that his or her immune system is underdeveloped and the gastrointestinal (G.I.) tract is not fully matured at birth. Colostrum's immune bioactives and growth factors are essential to encourage immune resilience and to complete the G.I. tract's maturation and development. All mammalian newborns have a "leaky gut" which is not only normal but beneficial – but only initially. The porous G.I. lining allows large proteins, such as immunoglobulins, to easily enter the bloodstream. Immunoglobulins in colostrum and mother's early milk bind to disease-causing pathogens on the mucosal surfaces of the G.I. tract, thereby preventing them from colonizing and causing infection.[11] This modulation by the immune system creates passive immunity for the infant – something that occurs in all mammals. Additionally, colostrum helps "seed" the newborn's G.I. tract by introducing beneficial bacteria into the microbiome. After getting this "jumpstart" from colostrum's immune bioactives, the growth factors go to work sealing up the porous G.I. lining so the gut is no longer leaky. The sealing up of the gut is in preparation for the arrival of breastmilk which gradually replaces the colostrum. Now, with a matured gut, milk will remain in the G.I. tract where it is digested into functional and absorbable nutrients, rather than seep into the bloodstream (where it's not supposed to be).

The maternal milk of all mammals offers passive protection to a newborn against enteric pathogens, and the historical concept of "immune milk" – the transfer of passive immunity via lacteal antibodies – dates back to the 1950s.[12] In the 1960s, the underlying mechanisms of passive immunity were realized when the chemical structure of immunoglobulins was discovered. Later in the 1970s, the secretory immune system was identified which gave way to the role of secretory antibodies in the prevention or treatment of enteric infections in mammals. Since the 1980s, there has been considerable interest in utilizing antibodies from the milk and colostrum of different mammalian species, particularly ruminants (i.e., cows and goats).

But let's step back a few decades to the 1940s so we can better understand why breastfeeding fell out of favor, so to speak. World War II was on, and large numbers of women were entering the workforce, so infant formulas provided a logical solution for infant feeding. After the war, successful marketing, coinciding with greater utilization of radio, television, and print advertising, resulted in a steady downward trend which continued through the 1950s and 1960s. By the early 1970s, 25% of infants were receiving breastmilk one week after birth and only 14% between two and 3 months of age.[13]

Kaye was born in the era of formula feeding, and we later learned that her mother never breastfed her at all. In retrospect, we believed that this was crux of her upper respiratory infections which set in motion the eventual radiation of her thymus gland by the family physician. Without the benefit of her mother's colostrum and milk, Kaye experienced successive infections. The dismal breast-feeding rates of the 1940s and 1950s seem to correlate with the more than 500,000 infants and children whose thymus was irradiated. On the other hand, my mother believed in breastfeeding her children and with eight of them, she had her hands full; my siblings and I have experienced exceedingly good health over the years without diabetes or autoimmune conditions. This, when taken into account the many individuals I personally know who were not breastfed, has bolstered my support for breastfeeding. Breastfeeding rates are on the rise again, but we can do better by removing or minimizing the impediments to breastfeeding.

IMPEDIMENTS to BREASTFEEDING
- Social norms (i.e. stigma of breastfeeding in public)
- Poor family and/or social support
- Maternal embarrassment regarding breastfeeding in public
- Hindrances resulting from a return to the workplace
- Lack of information about the benefits of breastfeeding
- Maternal lactation problems (i.e., sore nipples, pain, leaking milk, mastitis, insufficient milk production)
- Infant lactation problems (i.e., failure to latch onto the breast)
- Infant was adopted

Studies show that bovine antibodies can be effective in the prevention or treatment of human diseases caused by enteropathogenic microbes (i.e., bacteria, viruses, protozoans, and fungi). Bovine colostrum is the most prevalent colostrum preparation available today, and it passes immunity to most of the disease-causing pathogens that the dairy cow has encountered in her lifetime, including the antibodies she received from her own mother. Interestingly, a cow can produce antibodies to a disease that it does not develop itself. For example, Dr. Albert Sabin used bovine colostrum to successfully treat polio and later isolated antibodies to create the first oral polio vaccine that helped eradicate polio.[14] The dairy cows were exposed to the polio virus simply by interacting with the polio-infected farmers and although cows don't get polio, antibodies will be expressed in their colostrum and milk. This makes cows a broad-spectrum, natural antibody-producing pharmacy – for human benefit, if we choose to drink their raw milk. Supplementing one's diet with powdered bovine colostrum may offer a potent source of antibodies on an ongoing basis – from childhood through adulthood. For comparison, bovine colostrum contains approximately 80% immune bioactives and growth factors, whereas raw bovine milk contains 1.5% – which is why raw milk is good, but colostrum is better.

Unfortunately, early weaning or exclusive formula use deprives the infant of the immunity provided by the mother who produces her own antibodies to various pathogens that she encounters. A lack of growth factors likely interferes with intestinal permeability and creates other gut-related issues. Thus, breastfeeding helps prevent childhood illnesses, such as colic, respiratory and ear infections, infectious diarrhea, food and airborne allergies, and can help prevent a re-emergence of leaky gut, which has been linked to autism,[15,16] type 1 diabetes,[17,18] and other autoimmune conditions. Breastfeeding not only helps prevent infectious diseases in infants, but research shows that longer breastfeeding is associated with better intellectual development through childhood and into adolescence.[19,20]

The bioactives in mother's colostrum and breast milk are vital to neurological development and just may make us smarter. A review of 17 breastfeeding/I.Q. studies showed that breastfed infants achieved a mean score of 3.44 points higher than non-breastfed infants; if the studies controlled for maternal I.Q., the mean score was a smaller benefit at 2.62 points.[21] A study of 468 full-term babies with follow-up from infancy through preschool concluded that additional months of exclusive breastfeeding (i.e., only breast milk) increased I.Q. score by as much as 5.45 points.[22] One study even suggests that a single month of breastfeeding increases I.Q. score at five years of age by three points.[23] Another study suggested that breastfeeding is associated with more favorable performance on intelligence tests 30 years later which in turn, may increase both educational attainment and income in adulthood.[24]

RISKS of NOT BREASTFEEDING*
- Acute otitis media
- Gastroenteritis
- Atopic dermatitis
- Severe lower respiratory infections
- Necrotizing enterocolitis
- Sudden infant death syndrome (SIDS)
- Type 1 diabetes
- Asthma
- Childhood leukemia
- In later life, higher risk of elevated blood pressure, obesity, type 2 diabetes, and autoimmune conditions

American Academy of Family Physicians. Breastfeeding, Family Physicians Supporting (position paper).

Two of the most common infectious and potentially dangerous conditions affecting infants and young children are gut-based diarrheal diseases and respiratory diseases. Diarrhea is especially lethal to infants and worldwide, it is the second leading cause of infant death from dehydration and anemia. In the U.S., rotavirus was the leading cause of severe diarrhea prior to 2006 when a rotavirus vaccine became available with the aid of dairy cows. Rotavirus is extremely contagious, and combined with low vaccination rates, accounts for outbreaks among both vaccinated and unvaccinated infants and young children in child care settings; the most severe cases involve unvaccinated children between the ages of three months and three years.[25] Rotavirus infections can also occur in the caregivers of infected children, immunocompromised individuals, and older folks – so this often means grandma and grandpa.

Likewise, bacterial gastroenteritis caused by *E. coli* or salmonella contaminated foods, can be deadly for infants and young children. Chronic diarrhea can lead to dehydration and electrolyte imbalance; if vomiting accompanies the diarrhea, it's much more difficult to prevent fluid loss. Typically, pediatricians tell parents to offer a sick child additional breast milk or an oral rehydration solution (i.e., Pedialyte®) to replace lost minerals including sodium and potassium. Studies with bovine colostrum have demonstrated the favorable activity against rotavirus,[26,27,28,29,30,31] as well as bacteria-induced gastroenteritis.[32]

Parasitic infections, such as cryptosporidiosis ("crypto"), are less common in the U.S. but can occur from ingesting feces-contaminated water from domestic lakes, streams, rivers, or swimming pools, from international travel, or from the diapers of an infected child. Once ingested, the parasites attach to and infect the epithelial cells of the ileum and colon. In HIV-exposed and HIV-positive children, cryptosporidiosis an opportunistic infection because the patient is already immunocompromised. Again, bovine colostrum studies have demonstrated improvement in severe cryptosporidiosis-associated diarrhea in young patients with and without HIV / AIDS.[33,34] Colostrum treatment also eliminated the parasite from the G.I. tract in a matter of weeks.

Infants, particularly those born prematurely, are most susceptible to infections of the lungs and respiratory tract because their lungs and immune systems are not fully developed.[35] Even in healthy, full-term infants, the first two years of life have the highest rate of infant mortality. In the absence of safe and effective vaccination, a variety of viral illnesses, including common colds, croup, bronchitis, respiratory syncytial virus (RSV), seasonal influenza, and more recently COVID-19 pose significant health risks. Viral infections typically go away within 10-14 days without treatment as the immune system mounts its defense against the virus, but this can seem like a lifetime when it comes to a vulnerable baby. A coexisting state of immunocompromise compounds the problem.

Bovine colostrum's potential use in pre-term, immunocompromised infants who don't receive enough of their mothers' colostrum or milk has sparked research studies using pre-term piglets;[36] benefits have been observed in instances of sepsis, necrotizing enterocolitis and neuroinflammation.[37,38] Follow-up human studies have shown feasibility in using bovine colostrum in the first few weeks of life to supplement mother's milk in preterm infants; the colostrum helps increase protein intake.[39] At the time of this writing, clinical trials with very preterm infants (less than 32 weeks gestation) are underway to determine the growth-promoting effect of bovine colostrum when used as a human milk fortifier.[40]

Giving lactoferrin (an immune bioactive in colostrum) as a preventative treatment in infants weighing less than 3.3 pounds helps prevent sepsis; it is even more effective in infants weighing less than 2.2 pounds.[41] Bovine colostrum supplementation has also been shown to be a useful way to help increase the weight of children with nonorganic failure to thrive.[42] Certainly, preterm infants should have their own mothers' colostrum, but if this isn't possible, bovine is the next best option. A powdered bovine colostrum supplement can be added to infant formula, dairy milk, yogurt, filtered apple juice or applesauce for easy ingestion at most ages.

Antibodies Identified in Bovine Colostrum May Offer Protection Against the Associated Disease/Condition:[43]

- *Bacillus cereus* – food poisoning
- *Campylobacter jejuni* – food poisoning
- *Candida albicans* – yeast infections; oral or topical thrush
- *Clostridium difficile* – food poisoning
- *Escherichia coli* – food poisoning; urogenital tract infections
- *Escherichia coli* O157:H7 – food poisoning; renal failure
- *Haemophilus influenzae* – respiratory infections; pneumonia; bacterial meningitis;
- *Helicobacter pylori* – stomach ulcers
- *Klebsiella pneumoniae* – pneumonia; urinary tract infections
- *Listeria monocytogenes* – food poisoning; meningitis; encephalitis; fetal death
- *Propionibacterium* acnes – acne
- *Salmonella enteritidis* – food poisoning
- *Salmonella typhimurium* – food poisoning
- *Staphylococcus aureus* – blood & skin infections, antibiotic resistant (MRSA)
- *Staphylococcus epidermis* – wound infections
- *Streptococcus agalactiae* – urogenital tract infections
- *Streptococcus mutans* – periodontal disease; heart infections
- *Streptococcus pyogenes* – strep throat; flesh-eating bacteria; kidney disease; blood poisoning
- *Yersinia enterocolitica* – food poisoning; sepsis

Since I mentioned infant formulas, I'll share my perspective, albeit an honestly harsh one, and a brief history of infant formula recipes. All formulas – past and present – are essentially "dead," and the earliest versions were basically "junk food for babies." Although they contain protein, fats, carbohydrates, vitamins, minerals, and more recently, lactoferrin and oligosaccharides, they contain none of the 1000+ living components present in either mother's milk or bovine colostrum supplements. Devoid of antibodies and immune-balancing bioactives, formulas simply cannot provide protection against disease-causing pathogens which attack an infant's immature immune system and G.I. tract. And without natural growth factors, formulas cannot promote optimal development of the body's many tissues. If formula is the only nutrition provided from day one, the newborn's leaky gut will remain leaky and the gut microbiome won't benefit from the diversity necessary to flourish.

The importance of good infant nutrition cannot be understated; the 20th century indeed witnessed significant improvements in infant health and decreased infant mortality rates. Prior to the "invention" of formula, a wet nurse would be employed if a new mother was unable to produce an adequate amount of breastmilk for her baby, had died in childbirth, or simply elected not to breastfeed. Wet nurses would feed their own child as well as the child in their care ("milk siblings"), or begin nursing the new child after weaning her own. The practice and profession of wet-nursing goes back as far as Ancient Rome and is also mentioned in various mythologies and the Bible. In the U.S., it was quite common for female slaves to breastfeed and care for the slave owners' children. Unfortunately, precious breast milk produced by enslaved women was prioritized for the white children of slave owners; children born into slavery received a mixture of cow's milk and dirty water, and many died as a result.[44] The importance of wet nurses should not be disregarded whether the practice was made by choice or by force – nor should the sacrifice by African-American families be forgotten. The historical effects stemming from slavery are theorized to be, in part, responsible for the racial disparity between white and black mothers in both breastfeeding and infant mortality rates.[45]

Wet-nursing became less common as formulas came in to existence in the latter part of the 19th century and early part of the 20th century. The first patented and marketed liquid formula in 1867 consisted of cow's milk, wheat flour, malt flour, and potassium bicarbonate; later it was sold as a powder. Other companies were quick to jump on the bandwagon, but many families could not afford the cost, so the consumption of commercial formulas was low. If an infant needed supplemental milk, boiled cow's milk was generally acceptable to European families, whereas American families were initially less accepting of "pasteurization" and preferred raw cow's milk. By the 1920s, evaporated milk was used for home-prepared formula, and in the 1930s and 1940s, evaporated milk (or cow's milk) plus water and corn syrup ("junk") were common. It wasn't until the 1950s and 1960s when commercially-prepared formula use overtook home-prepared formula in the interest of convenience over cost considerations. Additionally, the formula industry and pediatricians heavily promoted its use to women as they entered the workforce in greater numbers.

Co-nursing – you might even call it modern day wet-nursing – is a similar practice characterized by reciprocal breastfeeding; it was and is more common among mothers who are siblings or close friends. Milk sharing for profit and milk donation have become more widely accepted practices today and seek to solve the problem of women not being able to produce enough breast milk. Another reason that the birth mother might not breastfeed is if it was medically contraindicated (i.e., she is HIV positive or uses illicit drugs).[46] Generally speaking, co-nursing and milk sharing came about because families realize the importance of breast milk as the best nutritional source an infant and toddler can receive. Human milk banks have been established around the world and are used by mothers who want a reliable milk source for their infants but have a low milk supply. These organizations carefully screen the donated milk, pasteurize it, and verify the health of the donors. Unfortunately, some mothers have resorted to using the Internet to arrange purchases of breast milk and that has turned out to be a risky practice. A 2013 study showed that, while good intentioned, 74% of breast milk samples purchased online contained infectious bacteria and 21% contained cytomegalovirus.[47] Additional data showed that 89% of the breast milk arrived above the recommended frozen temperature.[48] In the interest of safety and lower cost, bovine colostrum presents a viable alternative and additive to commercially available formula or a mother's own low milk supply.

Whether misguided doctors or a greedy formula industry or some combination, formula use put millions of children around the world at a disadvantage. Mothers were sold the idea that formula was superior to their own free breast milk. What mother doesn't want the absolute best for her child? Ironically, it was often wealthier families that could afford infant formula, and so their babies received the least amount of colostrum and breast milk, if any at all. In the last part of the 20th century, breastfeeding was on the rise, as was formula use with a decrease in feeding of cow's milk. This reversal likely emerged due to negative publicity towards the formula industry for their aggressive – and unethical – formula marketing to mothers in third world countries. The use of synthetic growth hormones and antibiotics in dairy cattle likely contributed to an aversion to bovine milk. The notion of *breast is best* has entered our collective consciousness and continues to influence rising breastfeeding rates. The science is catching up...or catching on, depending how you look at it.

I want to end this chapter with a final thought: Colostrum and milk are the perfect foods that intimately connect us to our mothers. When an infant nurses at mom's breast or a calf suckles its mother's teats, that young life is drinking life itself. These mammary secretions are "alive" and they become part of the infant, calf, and every other living being that breastfeeds. Ancient Egyptians believed that milk from the cow goddesses granted magical powers to the pharoah – life, power, wisdom, divinity, and renewal. Our children probably won't grow up to be rulers, but let us at least provide the life-giving and life-renewing qualities of colostrum and breast milk to help them thrive in life.

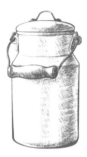

> ❝
> Look at those animals and remember
> the greatest scientists in the world have
> never discovered how to make grass into milk.
> *Michael Idvorsky Pupin*
> ❞

3

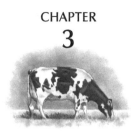

Dead Milk and Declining Health in Western Civilizations

In slower, simpler times, we received our milk from the local dairy that delivered it fresh to our doorstep every morning or every few mornings. And, yes, I am dating myself, so perhaps this experience was one of your parents' or grandparent's generation. What an excellent time to pick up the phone and give Mom or Dad a call to inquire about their local milkman. The time from cow's udder to our icebox (the refrigerator) was often a matter of hours rather than days, and the milk was often unpasteurized. Since iceboxes were literally boxes with blocks of ice in them, you couldn't keep the milk very long, so you tended to drink it rapidly and before the next delivery. Milk was typically drunk at most meals, since soda and other sugary beverages were not as common as today and consumed as treats or special occasion beverages, not dietary staples.

Nowadays, milk is produced in enormous dairies where the milk from thousands of cows is processed and pasteurized before being shipped to grocery or club stores. Once there, it may sit for weeks in cold storage before customers pick up a half gallon and bring it home, and again, it may sit another few weeks before being consumed entirely. Certainly, there's no question that modern dairies are models of efficiency and cleanliness, but there's a rather significant problem – milk produced by these dairies is as dead as roadkill. Any beneficial bacteria that had once been in it are killed by the pasteurization process, and virtually all of the beneficial proteins are denatured and rendered biologically useless. Pasteurized milk serves only one real purpose – to be a source of calories, amino acids, some vitamin D and calcium. In other words, REAL® milk is really "useless" from an immune resiliency standpoint compared to raw, fresh milk. Henceforward, I'll refer to what's sold in stores as "dead milk."

You may be asking yourself, what about all the naysayers who claim that milk, butter, cheese, steaks, and hamburgers are bad for you? I agree to some extent, but only if the cattle are conventionally raised and the milk is ultra-pasteurized and homogenized. Otherwise, I believe that pasture-raised meats and dairy foods have a place in one's daily diet so long as they are consumed in moderation. Foods derived from pasture-raised animals are typically higher in omega-3 fatty acids and conjugated linoleic acid while simultaneously lower in pro-inflammatory omega-6 fatty acids. This is due to the natural grasses they graze upon, and the beneficial effect for meat-eaters is less inflammation in the body than when derived from grain-fed animals.

Having been raised on a farm myself, one might expect me to be a proponent of dairy and meat. While I respect anyone's decision to be vegetarian or vegan, I do not believe it to be a nutritional choice that promotes optimal health. In this regard, it comes back to the concept of "living milk" and colostrum. Supplementing with bovine colostrum is ideal for vegetarians, and I'll address the rationale later in this chapter.

Raw milk has long been known to contain beneficial enzymes, growth factors, immunoglobulins and other proteins and peptides that can benefit humans of any age. For babies, the advantages of feasting on mother's milk as opposed to formula have been well-documented as detailed in Chapter 2. Breastfed babies are generally healthier than non-breastfed babies because they drink mom's "living milk" rather than "dead milk," or formula. Formula contains macronutrients such as fat, protein, and carbohydrates and micronutrients such as vitamins, minerals, and more recently oligosaccharides and lactoferrin, but it's absolutely nothing like what comes fresh from a mother's breast. Mother's milk is biologically active, or as I say…"alive." Formula sits in a canister on a grocery store shelf and it's as dead as a doornail.

The same is true of milk sourced from cows. If it has been over pasteurized – as nearly all commercial milk has been – it is essentially "dead." It retains no or very low biological activity. Conversely, living cow's milk – milk that has been pasteurized in such a way as to kill pathogens without significantly affecting its biological activity – retains some of the benefits of natural proteins and peptides found in milk. Unfortunately, our understanding of the importance of why we should drink milk has been reduced to calcium, vitamin D and strong bones. Living milk is so much more than that, and of course, raw, fresh cow's milk is the ultimate living milk, the same way mom's breastmilk is.

In order to understand the importance of consuming bioactive milk and milk products, we need to look at our common history with the cow. The relationship between man and bovine is one of the longest in our historical existence. Even before the development of agriculture and animal husbandry which allowed humans to live in one place, there was human-bovine interaction. Paleolithic drawings from the last Ice Age between 10,000 and 40,000 years ago show a growing dependence on the aurochs, an extinct species of wild cattle that inhabited North Africa, Asia, and Europe. According to medical anthropologist John Heinerman, Ph.D., it is likely that primitive humans used the aurochs not just as a source of meat but also milk and colostrum. Domestic cattle descended from the aurochs at a time when humans became more civilized.

The interdependent relationship between humans and domesticated animals extended to cattle, and as people settled down on farms and planted food crops, this relationship became even more intimate. Often, people would share their dwellings with their cattle or goats to protect them and keep them warm in harsh winter climates. In doing so, there was a readily available source of food in the form of milk and colostrum. As a consequence – or perhaps, a benefit – the infectious diseases of cows and goats were often shared with their human cohabitants, and vice versa. Thus, the immune protection offered by the milk and colostrum became important to the human family's health as well. This symbiotic relationship benefitted everyone in the household – children and adults alike – for as long as the cow or goat was milked.

Once the cows and other ruminant milk-producing animals moved out of the house, they were still close by – in a barn or nearby pasture – and they continued to provide raw, fresh milk every day for the family. The "living milk" was the dietary focal point, and the immune bioactives and growth factors were plentiful. Yet as people left the family farm and moved to urban centers, their diets changed greatly, and the close link to the milk-producing animal was broken. Modern dairy technology dramatically changed both the physical properties and health benefits of milk. The mass production and widely available pasteurized, homogenized milk and other dairy products all but guaranteed the disappearance of the critical immune bioactives and growth factors we once depended on. And with this disappearance came the emergence of allergies, autoimmune diseases, and other chronic health conditions. Of course, the development of processed and nutrient-deficient foods didn't help either.

Pasteurization is the process of heating milk and other dairy products in order to kill pathogenic bacteria with the intention of preventing foodborne illnesses. That seems reasonable, but heat also denatures proteins, deactivates beneficial enzymes, vitamins, growth factors, immune bioactives, and destroys the good bacteria that are naturally present in the milk. Maybe you're asking yourself, *why is this all necessary and why are we concerned about cow's milk but not human milk?* Cow's milk is susceptible to feces being splashed upwards onto the cow's udder while she is being milked, thereby potentially contaminating the milk; obviously, this is not the case with nursing mothers. Hundreds or thousands of cows are milked together, so any one of them could be a potential source of *E. coli* or other bacterial contamination. To ensure the milk supply is safe for consumers – some of whom may be immunocompromised – milk is pasteurized and thus rendered a "dead" food.

Spoiler Alert: I just described an outdated rationale. Today's milk collection processes are extremely modern and sanitary – from the moment the cow walks into the sterilized milking parlor. Her udders are thoroughly cleansed and tail pinned up as she stands on an elevated platform (i.e., no splashed feces); the automated milking apparatus is applied to her teats without her ever being touched by human hands. The milk is transferred to sterile containers where it is chilled to prevent bacteria growth and continually mixed to prevent separation... and eventually, it goes on to be pasteurized. But with such sanitary collection and storage processes, there's no rational reason to pasteurize it into a "dead" food.

To myself and many others, it's simply vexing, but we realize it's unlikely to change. This is why I advocate for the consumption of raw milk and its "living" qualities. Depending upon where you live, it may be difficult to locate raw milk, yogurt, kefir, or cheese for purchase because the consumption of raw, unpasteurized milk is subject to federal and state law.

For a historical perspective, milk pasteurization was slow to catch on in the United States following its development by microbiologist and chemist Louis Pasteur in 1864 who was ironically, attempting to lengthen the shelf life of his favorite wine.[48] Chicago was the first U.S. city in 1908 to require dairies selling milk within the city limits be pasteurized. The U.S. Public Health Service (later part of the Food and Drug Administration) established the Standard Milk Ordinance (SMO) in 1924 as guidance for state and local milk producing agencies. The SMO was voluntary and subject to agency interpretation, so in 1927, an ordinance code was added to ensure satisfactory compliance. The document and code were updated over the years and by the late 1940s, all milk sold to U.S. consumers required pasteurization. In 1965, the document was renamed "Grade A Pasteurized Milk Ordinance" (PMO). The current revision of the PMO was issued in 2017 and is available online.[49]

Don't get me wrong, pasteurization was valuable technology in the late 1800s and early 1900s. Not only was tuberculosis (TB) rampant at the time, but easily spread through contaminated milk. This occurred when a TB-positive worker coughed and respiratory droplets got into the milk pail. Prior to pasteurization, TB-contaminated milk was distributed within the community, infecting milk drinkers who could then spread their infection to others.

The U.S. Food and Drug Administration (FDA) bans the sale and/or distribution of raw milk across state lines. Drinking raw milk is legal in all fifty states, but individual states set their own laws regarding raw milk sales. As of 2016, thirteen states were allowed to sell raw milk in stores; seventeen allowed raw milk sales directly on the farm; and twenty states prohibit all raw milk sales.[50] If you live in a state that prohibits the sale of raw milk and your neighbor has a cow in his backyard, he can of course, *share* a glass with you. If you want to learn more about the benefits of raw milk, I suggest you look into the Weston A. Price Foundation (westonaprice.org). They are an advocacy group that promotes local farmers and traditional foods including pastured meats and raw milk.

Local farmer's markets and CSA (community sponsored agriculture) groups often offer raw milk dairy products. These smaller scale farming operations follow safe food practices just like the bigger farms and perhaps even more so because of their dedication to their local customers. Their products are not just commodities. Farmers believe in the health-promoting benefits of raw dairy and want to continue sharing this gift with others. Whether you choose raw milk at your local farmer's market or pasteurized milk from the grocery store, you will be a better consumer if you know the different types of pasteurization utilized in the industry.

Most milk is pasteurized by heating it to 161°F for fifteen seconds (sometimes called flash pasteurization) and then rapidly cooled. It can also be heated slowly to 145°F and held at that temperature for thirty minutes (sometimes called batch or vat pasteurization). Either method kills most of the harmful bacteria that could potentially make you ill. Any surviving bacteria will be kept in check (won't multiply) by keeping the milk refrigerated at 45°F or lower. This type of milk is what you'll find in the refrigerated section at the store; it has a relatively short shelf life, especially once you've opened it.

In comparison, ultra-pasteurization, designated UP (sometimes called super-pasteurization) entails heating the milk to at least 280°F for no less than two seconds. The high heat of ultra-pasteurization kills absolutely all life in the milk – it's "double dead" milk. Taking it a step further, ultra-high temperature pasteurization (UHT) utilizes a heating temperature of between 275°F and 300°F. Both UP processes allow for milk to be boxed and sit unrefrigerated on store shelves with a much longer expiration date.

Milk pasteurization is a fact of life especially for urban dwellers who do not have access to a local farmer's market or CSA. After milk pasteurization became mandatory in the late 1940s, urban areas experienced a significant decline in the spread of infectious diseases and infant mortality. This may be attributable to higher standards of cleanliness and reduced contamination in food processing facilities and improvements in overall hygiene. There's no doubt that it has prevented countless food-borne infections and reduced the incidence of acute kidney failure and death, especially in immunocompromised individuals.

The issue of pasteurization came up rather quickly when I was researching colostrum processing methods since colostrum for human consumption is covered by the PMO. Farmers were more than willing to give me their excess liquid colostrum for Kaye, but it only lasted a few weeks in the refrigerator before spoiling. So, like my colleague who'd reminded me about colostrum, I began drying it with a food dehydrator. This small-scale operation in our kitchen certainly wouldn't do if we were ever to "go big." I needed a viable preservation method that also took into account the logistics of collection from the dairies and temporary storage until the actual processing. Ensuring that colostrum's bioactives remained "living" in the end-product was paramount. Kaye thrived on our homemade powdered colostrum, but as I began experimenting on a much larger scale with various pasteurization and drying techniques, I initially stumbled. The batch method of slowly heating the colostrum in a vat and holding it at a specific temperature for thirty minutes or longer destroyed the living bioactives. When Kaye took this colostrum, her symptoms would return within a few days, so I literally needed my wife to tell me whether I was doing it right or not.

Lengthy cooking times, even at moderate temperatures, seemed to be the most significant contributors to colostrum ineffectiveness. We also found this to be true for commercially available, veterinary-grade colostrum supplements that were on the market at the time. Kaye was the ultimate test subject…like the canary in the coal mine when it came to validating colostrum's effectiveness. Everything Kaye's body was telling us fueled our knowledge and guided us towards developing a pure, safe, stable, and effective colostrum supplement that we could make available on a massive scale for millions of people who needed it.

Flash pasteurization did not destroy the bioactives and so, that was one problem solved. However, pasteurization isn't the only modern processing method that changes the natural properties of raw milk. Homogenization is also widely employed in commercial milk production, and I believe it further contributes to "dead milk" and may actually cause an allergic reaction. While pasteurization is designed for milk safety, homogenization is designed for milk consistency and taste. In its natural state, whether pasteurized or not, milk separates after some time; the fat molecules rise to the top to form a layer of cream. You could simply shake or stir the milk to return it to the consistency as it came out of the cow, but in time, it would separate again. Homogenization is a mechanical process that permanently prevents separation by breaking down the fat molecules so small that they remain evenly distributed throughout the milk.

Additional advantages include being able to combine milk from thousands of cows into one batch and increasing shelf-life. Proponents also say that homogenized milk is visually more appealing as a uniform white liquid, but obviously, that all depends on what one is accustomed to drinking. Homogenized milk wasn't popular until the

1920s, more than two decades after the invention of the emulsifying machine (the Gaulin Homogenizer) by French inventor Auguste Gaulin. In fact, consumers didn't believe this new type of milk was good for them until some persuasive marketing convinced them that homogenized milk was better for digestion.

To the contrary, I believe that the mechanical process of homogenization is detrimental in the context of leaky gut. In the pursuit of making the fat molecules smaller, the Gaulin Homogenizer uses high pressure to force all of the milk through hair-like tubes. Inevitably, the milk proteins are made smaller and as such, may readily pass though the tight junctions of a leaky gut, thereby gaining access to the bloodstream. Once in the bloodstream, the immune system is likely to mount an inflammatory reaction to these "foreign molecules." Over time, this could precipitate a milk allergy or sensitivity. More research is needed to confirm my suspicions. Fortunately, bovine colostrum that is made into a shelf-stable powdered supplement doesn't require homogenization. It is flash pasteurized to maintain maximum bioavailability and effectiveness while eliminating any potential pathogenic contamination.

At this point, here's my question to readers: *Has this discussion of pasteurization and homogenization given you pause to think differently about the milk you drink, or the milk you don't drink?* I'm not saying you need to run out to your local farmer's market to get raw, non-homogenized milk, but I encourage you to broaden your horizons and look beyond that which is familiar. And by the way, I've primarily talked about cow's milk. Milk from other ruminant animals is increasingly more available – goat, sheep, camel, and bison – well, maybe not bison – it would be an understatement to say they're a bit temperamental (or downright mean).

As Americans became more disconnected from life on the family farm, successive generations became disconnected from the knowledge of where food itself comes from – the very food that sustains all of us. In 2018, family farmers and ranchers comprised less than 2% of the U.S. population,[51] whereas when the U.S. was first settled, nearly everyone had a direct connection to agriculture and animal husbandry. Simply put, if you didn't grow it in your backyard, you didn't eat. Today, surveys show that the disengagement is not the only problem; misinformation about food is also problematic among much of the American public.[52] A 2017 online survey commissioned by the Innovation Center of U.S. Dairy reported that 7% of American adults believe that brown cows produce chocolate milk.[53] To put that in stark terms, more than sixteen million milk-drinking adults – not children – are misinformed about what comes out of cows and could not make chocolate milk from scratch.

When society becomes disconnected from its natural roots, health suffers. We need look no further than the explosion of chronic disease in Western countries. The Centers for Disease Control and Prevention (CDC) estimates that six in ten American adults have a chronic disease and four in ten have two or more chronic diseases.[54] Most physicians agree that nearly every American will die of a preventable autoimmune disease, whether heart disease, cancer, diabetes, lung disease, depression, or Alzheimer's disease. This is quite a big contrast to just a mere century ago. Although life expectancy was shorter in those days, your grandparents or great grandparents would have known very few people with any major chronic disease. Their friends, neighbors, and family members would have been more likely to die from an infectious disease such as smallpox, polio, or influenza. The period of suffering would have been significantly shorter – days, weeks, or months, not years or decades.

Today, not only do more people have multiple chronic

diseases, but these diseases are occurring at an earlier age. And thanks to modern medicine, people are living with the disease for many decades, so the period of suffering is significantly longer. For example, type 2 diabetes was once a disease that only developed in mid-life and beyond; now, with obesity on the rise, youngsters are developing the disease at an alarming rate. Living an additional two to three decades with diabetes increases the risk of complications due to disease progression; despite new pharmaceutical drugs to treat diabetes, the "wear and tear" is undeniably cumulative.

Many autoimmune and chronic diseases have their roots in poor nutrition – eating processed (dead) foods devoid of any biologic benefit and the toxic nature of the environment in which those foods were grown. Therefore, good nutrition is perhaps our best strategy to tackle this problem, and living foods such as vegetables and fruits (organic, if possible), minimally processed grains, pastured meats, and dairy products from pasture-raised cows and goats are a great place to start. Reconnecting with the source of our ancient health through milk and colostrum are vital to immune resiliency. Failure to act dooms us and our children to shorter lives plagued by chronic diseases of increasing severity and debility while traditional medicine looks on from the sidelines growing rich by pushing pharmaceutical band-aids. It's our choice and our responsibility to solve the problem.

So how do we get some of that good ol' fashioned dairy feeling? Short of buying fresh milk from the farm and drinking it unpasteurized – I won't even try to convince the detractors – is to supplement one's daily diet with bovine colostrum. When processed properly, colostrum is the best natural source of all that's missing from dead milk. And a final word to my vegetarian friends and "nut-milk" drinkers: The immune bioactives and growth factors that are essential for immune resiliency and optimal health are ONLY found in mammalian milk and colostrum, and colostrum, by far, has more of these components than either raw or pasteurized milk. Furthermore, I consider colostrum to be a unique food unto itself – less of an animal food per say – and more of immune sustenance and the "gift of life" from mother to child. In India, the cow represents Mother Goddess and is revered by Hindus as a symbol of the earth's bounty. Bovine colostrum is Mother Earth's bounty and will help us reclaim health in Western civilizations if we choose.

66

PRPs are probably the most significant natural substances in the human body relating to the immune system. Taking theses peptides as we age, we redirect our bodies to function in homeostasis.

Andrew Keech, Ph.D.

99

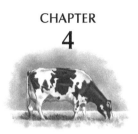

Colostrum:
Regulate. Repair. Regenerate.

A mother's colostrum and milk are biologically active, or "alive" as I've said, and will continue to remind readers throughout this book. This is such an important concept because we, as living beings, can benefit tremendously. It is my firm belief that colostrum is at least the SUM of its parts, and perhaps, SOME more. The immune bioactives, growth factors, and other nutrients – many of which have been identified and others that remain a mystery – work synergistically with each other. Exactly how this synergy coalesces also remains a mystery. Yet, like anything that is considered health-enhancing, it elicits man's desire to identify and isolate that unique component (or components) – one that can be made into a patentable and profitable drug. Colostrum itself is non-patentable, in the same way that a nutritious, non-GMO carrot is non-patentable. That is not to say that pharmaceutical companies have not isolated specific components and used them as the basis for drugs or stand-alone dietary supplements. But with so much wonderful "stuff" in colostrum, it makes infinite sense to take it whole, rather than in parts.

I must caution you that the next few pages – and even the next chapter – are going to get a little heavy on the science of colostrum. So, here's a visual depicting the most significant components which contribute to the life-giving and health-enhancing qualities of bovine colostrum (*See Figure 2*). By familiarizing yourself with these terms, you'll be ahead of the game, as these are some which appear frequently in the scientific literature and consumer publications.

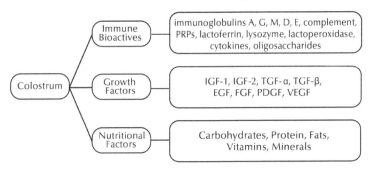

Figure 2: Most Significant Components in Colostrum

Researchers once believed that immunoglobulins were the most important components, primarily because these were one of the first type of component that they were able to identify and measure in colostrum samples. Farmers probably understood the benefits of immunoglobulins well before the scientists; they knew that if their newborn calves and foals did not receive colostrum from their mothers, they would die of infections shortly after birth. This intuitive knowledge was passed on from generation to generation while people lived on farms and participated in the lifecycle of the animals they raised. Colostrum's immunoglobulins are excellent for preventing gut-based infections, and the scientific literature has well documented this.

There is something to be said for humans' observation and assessment of the natural world, even if the scientific evidence is lacking. Anecdotal accounts of colostrum's healing qualities are direct observation of phenomena within a natural setting, the very definition of observational research. As I note in the account of Kaye's health transformation, we did not know what was in colostrum that made it effective;

we just knew that it was effective. All of colostrum's healing components are present in a state of natural balance and are not found in any other foods, except in small quantities in raw fresh milk.

Approximately 250 individual components in colostrum have been identified to date, yet there are likely over one-thousand, with many of these being represented as specific antibodies and no fewer than 600 polypeptides. Below is a list of the most prevalent components – categorized as either *immune bioactives* or *growth factors* – and a brief description. *(See Appendix A for a more comprehensive list.)* Certainly, as we develop new technologies to analyze the composition of colostrum, the list will expand. I encourage readers to utilize Wikipedia (wikipedia.org) and/or PubMed (pubmed.ncbi.nlm.nih.gov) to learn more about their biological functions within the human body. I list the ones that have been determined to exert the most impact on health, and I'll begin with the immunoglobulins.

IMMUNE BIOACTIVES

Immunoglobulins (antibodies) are large protein chains that mammals produce and use to recognize and bind antigens (foreign substances); they identify and mark viral or bacterial cells for destruction. Immunoglobulins in bovine colostrum bind to disease-causing pathogens on the mucosal surfaces of the gastrointestinal (G.I.) tract, thereby preventing them from colonizing and causing infection. Immunoglobulins are classified into five broad groups (i.e., IgG, IgA, IgM, IgE, IgD). Immunoglobulin G and immunoglobulin A are the most critical in regards to immune protection. Only IgG is transferred via the placenta in humans. IgA, IgM, IgE, and IgD are solely expressed in the offspring's body.

IgG is the immunoglobulin most abundant in bovine colostrum and the most common immunoglobulin circulating within human body. IgG is produced in the white blood cells of bone marrow and carried into the blood and lymph system whereby it identifies and neutralizes specific viruses, bacteria, and associated toxins. In humans, IgG is transferred from mother to fetus via the placenta but in cows, IgG is transferred to a great extent through colostrum. This is why bovine colostrum is noted for its high IgG content – between 70 – 80% of the total bovine immunoglobulins in raw colostrum. In cows, IgG provides systemic immunity.

There are four sub-classes of immunoglobulin G – IgG1, IgG2, IgG3, and IgG4; sub-classes 1 and 2 are the most abundant. IgG1 is important in the immune response to viral pathogens. IgG2 defends against bacteria that are encapsulated in a polysaccharide (complex sugar). IgG3 affects the immune response to protein antigens. The role of IgG4 remains a bit of a mystery.

IgA has potent, broad-based antiviral and antibacterial abilities by which it helps prevent infection, particularly of the respiratory tract, G.I. tract, and genitals. The most abundant form of IgA is found in mucous secretions such as saliva, tears, and sweat, and colostrum; a less abundant form is found in blood serum. The transfer of IgA through breastfeeding is highly efficacious in preventing respiratory and gutbased infections in human infants. IgA comprises between 10 – 15% of the total bovine immunoglobulins in raw colostrum.

IgM is produced in the spleen and appears when an antigen is initially detected; its involvement in the early phase of an infection makes it a useful test in the determination of a current or previous infectious disease. IgM comprises between 10 – 15% of the total bovine immunoglobulins in raw colostrum and has strong anti-bacterial activity.

IgE binds to receptors on mast cells to help modulate the allergenic response (i.e., release of histamine) in conditions such as asthma, allergic rhinitis, atopic dermatitis, food allergies, and various allergens that can cause anaphylaxis (i.e., bees stings, insect bites, medications). IgE also provides immunity to protozoan parasites and their venom. IgE's abundance is relatively low both in the human body and in raw bovine colostrum, but it packs quite a punch to create a massive inflammatory reaction to destroy an antigen.

IgD has robust antiviral activity, is found in small quantities in blood serum, and is often expressed along with IgM. Raw bovine colostrum contains only small quantities of IgD.

Species	Immunoglobulin	Concentration and (% of total immunoglobulins) Colostrum	Concentration and (% of total immunoglobulins) Milk
BOVINE	IgG_1	47.60 mg/mL (81.0%)	0.59 mg/mL (73.0%)
	IgG_2	2.90 mg/mL (5.0%)	0.02 mg/mL (2.5%)
	IgA	3.90 mg/mL (7.0%)	0.14 mg/mL (18%)
	IgM	4.20 mg/mL (7.0%)	0.05 mg/mL (6.5%)
HUMAN	IgG	0.43 mg/mL (2.0%)	0.04 mg/mL (3.0%)
	IgA	17.35 mg/mL (90.0%)	1.00 mg/mL (87%)
	IgM	1.59 mg/mL (8.0%)	0.10 mg/mL (10%)

SOURCE: Butler, J. E. Synthesis and distribution of immunoglobulins. *J. Am. Vet. Med. Assoc.* 1973. 163:795–798.

Table 1: Immunoglobulins in Bovine and Human Colostrum & Milk[55]

Complement is a group of more than thirty proteins that work together to eliminate pathogenic microorganisms from the body's tissues and blood. The complement system (C3) achieves this by "complementing" the action of antibodies and phagocytic cells. This includes (1) attacking the pathogen's cell membrane, causing lysis; (2) removing damaged cells and cellular debris; and (3) promoting inflammation of the surrounding tissue. Proteins in the complement system are primarily produced by the liver and circulate in an inactivated state in the bloodstream; when an activation signal is received, indicating the presence of a pathogen, C3 comes online through a series of chemical reactions to eliminate the "foreign invader."

Lactoferrin is an iron-binding protein with an arsenal of microbe-killing mechanisms, including depriving pathogenic bacteria of the iron it needs to reproduce itself during an infection. Lactoferrin also competes with pathogens for binding sites on the intestinal wall or binds directly to the outer membrane of viruses, bacteria, and fungi to lyse (burst) them. It is also an essential growth factor for lymphocytes (white blood cells) and increases natural killer (NK) cell activity. Lactoferrin modulates the immune system by stimulating cytokine (signaling molecules) production which in turn, promotes or inhibits inflammation during an infection. Aside from its immunoregulatory action, lactoferrin helps maintain the body's iron balance and regulate bone metabolism.

Lactoferrin's many applications have somewhat recently garnered increased attention, and after the FDA deemed it to be a safe food supplement, its use has increased. Whether extracted from bovine colostrum or manufactured with recombinant DNA technology, lactoferrin is now used as either a stand-alone dietary supplement or as an additive to other foods. The benefits for infant intestinal health and reducing gut-based pathogens has propelled lactoferrin's use in infant formulas. Because lactoferrin prevents viruses from attaching to target cells, it offers promise for combatting common infections including colds, flu, gastroenteritis, and herpes.[56] Its various modes of action are also useful in addressing cancerous tumors, and by optimizing the immune system, lactoferrin has a role in preventing cancers of the tongue, esophagus, lungs, bladder, and colon.[57]

Lysozyme is an enzyme that damages the cell membrane of bacteria which results in lysis (bursting). Lysozyme often works in tandem with lactoferrin, and they are particularly effective against diarrheal disease in young children.

Lactoperoxidase is an enzyme that when it combines with

various substrates and hydrogen peroxide (naturally present in the human body), forms a potent antibacterial agent.

Oligosaccharides are complex sugar molecules that exist alone or attached to amino acids (glycoproteins) or lipids (glycolipids). They compete with bacterial pathogens for binding sites on the cells that line the G.I. tract; in doing so, oligosaccharides prevent pathogens – often *E. coli* – from attaching to the gut wall and entering the bloodstream. In newborns, oligosaccharides provide protection in the first few days in the life when they are most susceptible to infections of the G.I. tract. Oligosaccharides also act as a prebiotic by promoting the growth of beneficial bacteria in the gut microbiome.

Proline-rich Polypeptides (PRPs) are short chains of peptides (proteins) with a high concentration of the amino acid proline. They are also called: info-peptides, info-proteins, cytokine precursors, and colostrinin. Basically, they modulate the immune system through a variety of mechanisms and support regulation of the thymus, the gland responsible for the normal development of immunologic function in the body. PRPs act as signaling molecules; induce white blood cell proliferation; modulate the cytokine system by stimulating the production of both pro-inflammatory cytokines (i.e., tumor necrosis factor-alpha and interferon-gamma), and the anti-inflammatory cytokines (i.e., interleukin-6 and interleukin-10).

The dual-function of PRPs is valuable depending on specific need. Some PRPs act against viral and bacterial pathogens by modulating the immune system to rally a defense against an infection, especially gut-based infections that cause massive diarrhea. PRPs increase the immune system's activity when it's necessary to fight off an infection. It does this by increasing inflammation; increasing lymphocyte and T-cell production and increasing natural killer cell activity to eliminate pathogens; and activating macrophages that devour the infected cells and cellular debris.

Other PRPs quell the immune system's activity to prevent tissue damage once the infection has been attenuated. It does this by decreasing inflammation; decreasing lymphocyte and T-cell production; decreasing natural killer cell activity; deactivating macrophages; and restoring normal cell function. Because PRPs are such a richly varied immune and inflammatory modulator, they are helpful in ailments characterized by an overactive immune system (allergies, asthma, and autoimmune diseases), including cognitive/neurodegenerative disorders. They can also tone down chronic low-grade inflammation which otherwise contributes to general unhealth.

Cytokines are small proteins that regulate the intensity and duration of the immune response, either by promoting inflammation or quelling inflammation. Cytokines mediate cell-to-cell communication, increase T-cell activity, and stimulate production of immunoglobulins. Sub-classes include interleukins and lymphokines. Colostrum contains various pro-inflammatory and anti-inflammatory cytokines and can also stimulate cytokine production in peripheral (in the bloodstream) blood cells. This leads to greater immune responsiveness, reduced infection severity, and return to immune homeostasis.

GROWTH PROMOTING FACTORS

Growth Factors are proteins or steroid hormones that act as signaling molecules between cells which play an important role in maintaining tissues, regeneration, and repair of damaged tissues within the human body. By stimulating cell growth, proliferation, differentiation and migration, growth factors (1) mature the newborn's leaky gut; (2) repair leaky gut in children and adults; (3) maintain or increase muscle, bone, tendon, and ligament tissue; (4) accelerate healing of injured or aging muscle, bone, cartilage, skin, nerves, and heart; (5) increase collagen production; (6) stimulate growth of blood vessels into damaged areas for increased circulation; (7) metabolize adipose tissue as a fuel source; and (8) balance blood glucose levels. Colostrum contains numerous growth factors, yet the most important ones include Insulin-like Growth Factor, Transforming Growth Factors, and Epithelial Growth Factor. Growth factor concentrations in colostrum are highest during the first few hours after the infant is born and decrease steadily in a time-dependent manner.

Insulin-like Growth Factor I (IGF-1) is a protein hormone with a molecular structure that is similar to insulin. IGF-1 is a major growth factor which affects nearly every type of cell, especially those in muscles, bones, connective tissue, nerves, lungs, kidneys, liver, and skin. IGF-1 assists with wound healing (i.e., bone fractures, cuts, scrapes, burns, muscle tears) by stimulating cell proliferation. Muscle injury, as elicited with resistance exercise and weight training, will in turn, increase muscle mass; this is the rationale for the interest in growth hormone (GH) and IGF-1 supplementation. IGF-1 production begins decreasing after puberty, and this steady decline through middle age into the latter years contributes to slower healing from injuries, immobility, and long-term bedrest. IGF-1 in mother's colostrum helps mature the newborn's G.I. tract.

Insulin-like Growth Factor II (IGF-2) is a protein hormone that functions similarly to IGF-1. It regulates the body's use of fat and protein. IFG-2 is a major fetal growth factor and promotes growth during gestation.

Transforming Growth Factor Alpha (TGF-α) is a cell signaling protein produced in keratinocytes (a type of skin cell), brain cells, macrophages, and within the cells of the stomach lining. The function of TGF-α is similar to EGF as it induces epithelial (skin) development. It can also stimulate neural cell growth following a brain injury.

Transforming Growth Factor Beta 1 & 2 (TGF- β1, TGF- β2) are cell signaling proteins produced by white blood cells that control cell growth, regeneration, differentiation, and apoptosis (cell death). TGF- β stimulates production of IgA by B-lymphocytes and is a vital factor in skeletal growth, bone mass maintenance, and fracture healing.

Fibroblast Growth Factors (FGF) are a family of cell signaling proteins that are important to wound healing. FGF stimulate blood vessel growth, stimulate cellular regeneration in wounds, help repair bone fractures, and maintain normal bone tissue. FGF's enhanced tissue repair capabilities also apply to burns, skin grafts, and ulcers.

Epithelial/Epidermal Growth Factor (EGF) are cell signaling proteins that stimulate the proliferation and differentiation of epidermal (skin) cells in the outer skin and those in the "inside skin" (intestinal lining). EGF is critical to maintaining gut integrity and normal permeability levels; thereby making it essential in combatting leaky gut.

Betacellulin belongs to the EGF family and since it has recently been identified, its function(s) is somewhat unclear. Betacellulin is believed to influence development of the neonatal gastrointestinal tract, and to regulate the differentiation of pancreatic beta cells during development and regenerate beta cells in adults. It has recently been suggested that betacellulin plays a role in various biological processes including reproduction, fluid homeostasis, and neural stem cell development.

Macrophage Colony Stimulating Factor (M-CSF) / Colony-Stimulating Factor-1 (CSF-1) stimulates stem cells in bone marrow to proliferate and differentiate into white blood cells, macrophages, and bone marrow progenitor cells. These cells help combat viral infections and clean up the cellular debris after the infection.

Granulocyte Colony Stimulating Factor (G-CSF) belongs to the colony stimulating factor (CSF) family that stimulates bone marrow to produce and activate granulo-cytes (eosinophils, basophils, neutrophils) and stem cells and release them into the bloodstream. G-CSF is helpful for immunocompromised states such as chemotherapy or radiation exposure where white blood cells have been depleted. G-CSF may also have neuroprotective properties.

Platelet-Derived Growth Factor (PDGF) plays a key role in blood vessel formation from existing vasculature (angiogenesis) and bone/osteoblast metabolism by regulating cell growth and cell division (mitogenesis). PGDF stimu-lates fibroblast division which assists in wound healing and ulcer healing. Its bone regeneration applications include periodontics, bone fractures, and orthopedic surgery.

Vascular Endothelial Growth Factor (VEGF) is a member of the platelet-derived growth factor (PDGF) family which stimulates angiogenesis in injured tissue and creates new blood vessels during embryonic development (vasculogenesis). VEGF helps heal injuries (i.e., muscles, tendons, ligaments) by enabling oxygen-rich blood to reach the damaged area or by creating collateral circulation to bypass blocked vessels.

OTHER IMPORTANT COMPONENTS & NUTRITIONAL FACTORS

Leptin is a hormone that suppresses appetite and helps increase energy expenditure and diminish fat storage. Suf-ficient or higher leptin levels may prevent overeating and weight gain.

Growth Hormone (GH) is an anabolic hormone which promotes muscle growth, fat mobilization, and inhibition of glucose utilization in favor of stored fat as a fuel source. GH in the body stimulates the production of IGF-1, which is the "real growth hormone."

Vitamins – B6, B12, Thiamine (B1), Riboflavin (B2), A, C, D, E, Folic Acid, Pantothenic Acid, Beta-carotene, Retinoic Acid

Minerals – Sodium, Calcium, Potassium, Magnesium, Chromium, Zinc, Chloride

Essential Amino Acids – Isoleucine, Leucine, Histidine, Methionine, Lysine, Threonine, Phenylalanine, Valine, Tryptophan

Non-Essential Amino Acids – Arginine, Cystine, Glutamic Acid, Alanine, Tyrosine, Glycine, Proline, Aspartic Acid, Serine

Fats – phospholipids, fatty acids, saposins, tocopherols, and cholesterol are present in whole colostrum. Because fats do not provide any significant benefit beyond infancy and also contribute to rancidity, they are frequently removed from bovine colostrum that is made into supplements.

Lactose is a sugar comprised of glucose and galactose. It is naturally present in whole colostrum but often removed when making supplements to help individuals with lactose sensitivity.

Macronutrient	Colostrum	Milk
Fat (%)	6.0–7.0	3.6–4.0
Protein (%)	14.0–16.0	3.1–3.2
Lactose (%)	2.0–3.0	4.7–5.0

Table 2: Macronutrient Content of Bovine Colostrum vs. Bovine Milk[58]

Whew! That's probably more information than you were expecting, but it illustrates just how complex colostrum is. More so, it provides the context for the immense interest – first by the dairy industry, then by others who sought to capitalize on the physiological, health-enhancing effects. From scientists to athletes to physicians to the pharmaceutical industry, the potential capabilities of the immune-modulating bioactives and growth-promoting factors in colostrum provided numerous applications. For everyday people like Kaye and myself, it was clear that colostrum possessed enormous potential as a nutritional supplement to improve health.

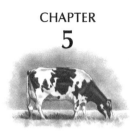

Colostrum Down Under

Up until this point on our journey, Kaye and I had our personal experience, the medical literature, but no real way to get beyond the limited amount of colostrum I could secure for Kaye's personal needs. If we ever hoped to make this amazing "gift of health" available to others on a massive scale, we would need some help...from above and from the other side of the globe.

Once we realized that our life path was pointing us in a new direction, a big, daunting, – and somewhat worrisome – question emerged. *How the heck do you produce a health food product from something that is considered a waste product?* The two seemed incompatible. So, I preferred to think of it as a once-in-a-lifetime challenge that would require a mix of out-of-the-box thinking, savvy salesmanship, persistence, and of course, some divine guidance. We, of course, already had a great story to tell – and some science for a foundation (so, no one would think we were crazy!) – and, everyone loves a heartwarming true story. There was never a dry eye after hearing Kaye tell her inspiring story.

Do you remember how I described colostrum as a dairy waste product in Chapter 1? Well, this was our first major hurdle in trying to create a viable product that could serve the needs of millions of people. In the early nineties, no one in the United States had much use for colostrum as a human consumable product. Animal feed was the only use, and even with that, most of the colostrum collected was simply discarded because there wasn't a large enough market for it. There was no feasible way to store fresh colostrum beyond a few weeks and no means to dry it on a massive scale. And keep in mind that colostrum wasn't considered milk, and any milk that contained colostrum could not be sold for human consumption. To top it off, the USDA's stringent standards for processing milk meant that you could not process colostrum in a facility that normally processed milk. Needless to say, Kaye and I were starting from behind the eight ball, and so began the process of bringing colostrum for human consumption to fruition.

The mission was simple: Find a way to improve colostrum collection at the dairy; process the colostrum so it would last more than two weeks without rendering it ineffective; and meet the safety standards for human consumption. Leaving colostrum in containers by the side of the road was obviously fraught with problems, particularly the potential for bacterial contamination. Fortunately, I was able to convince dairy farmers to store their excess colostrum in freezers until it could be picked up, and that bought me more time to collect the colostrum without it spoiling, as well as experiment with different processing methods. Even more important was finding dairy companies that would process the colostrum for me using the high-quality standards for milk processing rather than the low-quality standards for animal-feed colostrum. Persistence paid off, and the dairies agreed to sterilize their processing equipment prior to running the colostrum through it. Otherwise, I would have simply been in the business of making colostrum for animal use.

Simultaneously, identifying an efficient drying process so that pasteurized, liquid colostrum could be turned into a shelf-stable powdered product was critical. This concept is akin to how powdered milk is made, but powdered milk is dried with high heat, which is problematic for colostrum's delicate components. High heat – from both pasteurization and drying – would destroy a large percentage of the immune bioactives and growth factors, and essentially create powdered milk (protein, carbohydrates, fat and some micronutrients) Additionally, animal-grade colostrum (in liquid form), would be sprayed through the hot air expelled by a gas flame. The burning of natural gas creates carcinogenic nitrates and these could be absorbed into the colostrum particles during the drying process. Thus, a new and safer drying method was needed.

As I experimented with various methodologies, I continued to generate enough colostrum for Kaye to maintain her immune system. Nailing down a standardization process was difficult in the beginning, and I didn't always get it right. Since heat is the biggest threat to colostrum's bioactives, an increase in the pasteurization or drying temperature could render the bioactives ineffective. Not getting it right meant that the colostrum did not work as well (or at all), and Kaye's symptoms would return. She'd catch a cold, be laid up for weeks, and I knew I'd failed us both. So, not only was Kaye my test subject, she was the canary in the coal mine, and my divine inspiration. With her guidance and support, I formed Symbiotics, Inc. in 1994.

The next few years presented a unique opportunity to get my fledgling colostrum company off the ground. One significant external event which influenced Symbiotics and every other health food company was the Dietary Supplement Health and Education Act of 1994, commonly known as DSHEA.[59] This legislation allayed public fear that the Food and Drug Administration (FDA) would ban the sale and use of dietary supplements, which had been debated in Congress in the late 1980s and early 1990s. DSHEA curbs the power of the FDA but sets forth regulations regarding the manufacture and sale of dietary supplements, including permissible product labeling claims. As with most legislation, there are critics and proponents, but I believe DSHEA has been good for Americans overall. It allows consumers to utilize natural substances that have been used throughout history (other than tobacco) if they choose for health purposes. Since DSHEA classifies dietary supplements as "not drugs," the Act places the burden of proof on the FDA to prove that such a product is unsafe.

Half-way around the globe and down under in the Southern Hemisphere, I discovered the New Zealand Dairy Group (NZDG). They were producing colostrum for human consumption in a way that I only dreamed of in the U.S. The pristine landscape, strict environmental laws, and lack of large-scale industrial polluters was ideal for raising and harvesting colostrum from "happy cows." New Zealand dairy farmers were savvy about their herds' natural antibody-generating potential, and colostrum analysis by an industry group proved them right. When compared to hyperimmune colostrum (i.e., cows intentionally inoculated), the non-hyperimmunized cows produced colostrum that contained naturally-induced antibodies to 19 specific pathogens that they tested (Refer to list in Chapter 2). It would have been next to impossible to test for all the antibodies because of the cost factor, but it's safe to say that the numbers would be in the range of the thousands. This now made bovine colostrum a valuable commodity for the natural health and nutrition marketplace. Incidentally, it also meant that human intervention (hyperimmunization) was not necessary – cows are the most perfect natural antibody factories all on their own.

At the time, NZDG produced the highest quality colostrum available worldwide, and in 1998, Symbiotics contracted with NZDG to produce colostrum for sale in the U.S. I intended to market colostrum as a nutritional supplement, but I was realistic about how it would take more than just putting a product on the shelf at a health food store to build up consumer acceptance and eventually, consumer demand.

While I spent time going back and forth between the U.S. and New Zealand, a like-minded soul was moving along a parallel path that would eventually come to intersect with mine. Two decades my junior, a young biochemist-in-the-making, Andrew Keech, Ph.D. was growing up on a New Zealand dairy farm. With experiences similar to mine on my grandfather's ranch, the young Andrew understood the importance of colostrum to the newborn calves. He excelled in school and went on to earn multiple degrees in mathematics, chemistry, and chemical and process engineering. Dr. Keech then put his knowledge to use as a protein biochemist/research engineer at the New Zealand Dairy Research Institute. I was introduced to Dr. Keech in 2003; shortly after, he moved to the U.S. to further his career. His commitment to unlocking the secrets of colostrum and the immune system was inspirational to Kaye and myself, and his years of research have benefitted the industry as a whole.

Interest in colostrum – derived primarily from sheep and cows – began to gain traction in the scientific community outside of the veterinary arena and dairy industry in the 1990s. This was likely due to an overall interest in discovering natural substances with applications for human health. The two primary "research camps" were gastrointestinal health and athletic enhancement. First, gastrointestinal infections such as rotavirus were common in developing nations where the lack of access to clean drinking water was widespread. Infants and young children are particularly susceptible to rotavirus, which causes massive diarrhea, leading to dehydration and death. Utilizing bovine colostrum as a treatment and method of passive immunization was viewed as a game-changer for improving infant health in areas where rotavirus was endemic.[60,61]

Second, the 1980s saw the emergence of HIV/AIDS which destroys the immune system and makes patients highly susceptible to G.I. and other opportunistic infections. Chronic diarrhea caused by *Cryptosporidium, Salmonella*, and cytomegalovirus infections were common, and although relatively easily eliminated by a healthy immune system, were not in an immunosuppressed individual. The inability to resolve the diarrhea and maintain nutritional uptake led to malnutrition, muscle wasting, and severe weight loss. Immunoglobulins from bovine colostrum were viewed as a potential neutralizing agent for bacterial, viral, and protozoan pathogens.[62] This research led to colostrum-based food supplements to treat HIV-associated diarrhea.[63,64,65] Nutritional approaches to G.I. infections are exceedingly valuable to developing countries where patients do not have access to or cannot afford expensive pharmaceutical drugs.

Third, there was great interest in whether bovine colostrum could serve as treatment and prevention for the damage to the intestinal lining caused by non-steroidal anti-inflammatory drug (NSAID) use, particularly by arthritis and chronic pain sufferers. The intestinal "injury," or permeability problems examined in these studies later became commonly known as "leaky gut" and was realized to be a widespread problem. It was not just NSAID users that developed leaky gut, but people who took other types of medications and substances which irritated and ulcerated the gut lining. The seminal research in this area was done by Raymond Playford, M.D., Ph.D., and he found colostrum to be effective as a natural remedy in addressing intestinal permeability.[66,67] An "ah ha" moment to come of this G.I.-related research was that bovine colostrum was a relatively inexpensive preventative that happened to be a food (not a drug), so you didn't need a physician's prescription to purchase it.

The other "research camp" – athletic enhancement – was also a natural fit for the clinical study of colostrum. In the early 2000s and as bovine colostrum became widely popular with athletes, consumer demand fueled the colostrum industry in the United States. Some early human trials of bovine colostrum supplementation involved competitive sports, as the high IGF-1 content was hypothesized to produce a performance-enhancing benefit in Olympic-level and professional athletes. In a world where performance is measured in milliseconds, any natural substance that enhances endurance and strength and reduces recovery time determines who wins the gold and who wins the silver. NZDG and Symbiotics helped introduce its New Zealand-sourced powdered colostrum to researchers at the University of Adelaide in Sydney, Australia who were investigating bovine colostrum's effect on athletic performance.

Athletes were the ideal market to target bovine colostrum; achieving that coveted performance edge without relying on an illegal or addictive substance was paramount. Synthetic human growth hormone (hGH) was on trend at the time, but obviously illegal, and later discovered to potentially contribute to cancer, joint pain, carpal tunnel syndrome, arm and leg swelling, glucose intolerance, increased risk of diabetes, and gynecomastia. On the other hand, the natural growth factors in bovine colostrum help burn fat, build lean muscle, build strength, shorten recovery time, balance blood glucose levels, prevent illness after vigorous exercise, reduce inflammation and pain, and even help prevent some types of cancer.

An interesting side story about Olympic athletes and colostrum: The International Olympic Committee (IOC) launched an inquiry into whether powdered bovine colostrum was a potentially banned substance following a higher than anticipated number of medals won by the Australian Olympic team in the 2000 and 2004 games.[68] The Australians claimed that their winning advantage was attributable to their athletes' colostrum supplementation during training.[69,70] The IOC determined that colostrum was instead a superfood, and their ruling provided athletes with a safe, viable, and legal alternative to doping and other banned substances. The World Anti-Doping Agency (WADA) continues to advise athletes against taking colostrum over unfounded concerns that it will increase plasma levels of IGF-1. Research published in 2020 concluded that supplementing with a standard colostrum dose (20-40 grams daily) did not cause circulating IGF-1 levels to increase either immediately or over time.[71] These findings support colostrum's safety profile, not just for athletes but anyone who desires to take advantage of the immune and G.I. health benefits.

In the 2010s, there was a fascinating crossover between the G.I. research and the athletic research when researchers discovered that intense exercise, such as that performed by elite athletes, made them susceptible to developing increased intestinal permeability. In extreme cases, heat stroke was partially attributable to transient leaky gut. Colostrum supplementation was able to truncate the increased intestinal permeability, thereby preventing heat stroke.[72] A later study showed that the addition of zinc carnosine (ZnC) enhanced the protective effect of colostrum and could be beneficial for military personnel as well as athletes.[73] This research suggests that colostrum, alone or in combination with ZnC, can facilitate the benefits of heavy exercise with less risk of heat stroke because exercise could continue unimpeded for a longer amount of time.

Because colostrum is not a standardized drug or even a standardized supplement, the obstacles in early colostrum research are much the same as today. There was significant variability in the origins (i.e., New Zealand, United States, Europe), the colostrum processing methods, the bioactives present, and the "dosing" (Remember: Colostrum is not a drug). Because of this, the results across human clinical studies varied widely, although most demonstrated a positive effect. Dosing in athletic clinical trials was typically 60 grams once or twice a day, and that was really the only consistency. This aspect of colostrum research is improving but will probably always vary somewhat because although cows will always produce colostrum, the immune bioactives and growth factor content will vary among different herds and individual cows. The good news is that what was once widely viewed as a waste product is now a profitable industry. However, at some point in the future, demand will outpace supply, especially if the overall demand for dairy milk decreases; fewer dairy cows used for milk production equals less colostrum output.

Of course, there have been some peaks and valleys in the colostrum industry over the last three decades. Initially, when word got out that colostrum was an all-natural performance-enhancing supplement, a lot of companies tried to cash in on colostrum's growing popularity. Eventually, cheaper, lower-quality colostrum supplements were brought to market. Even an educated colostrum consumer had little to no knowledge of the significance pasteurization methods or milk dryer heat, so when an athlete or body builder stopped getting the benefits they had been getting previously, they simply stopped buying colostrum. Many chalked it up to colostrum being a nutritional fad that just stopped working, and as you'd expect, sales plummeted.

Another reason for the decline in sales was a significant drop in the efficacy of New Zealand colostrum. In 2001, NZDG merged with Kiwi Cooperative Dairies and the New Zealand Dairy Board to form Fonterra, the single largest dairy company in New Zealand. The merger may have been good for independent dairy farmers, but it was disastrous for colostrum. Fonterra pooled together all the colostrum and dried it in huge milk driers – the same driers used to make powdered milk. The high heat of the milk driers rendered the colostrum essentially useless. So, in an odd turn of events, the misguided decision in New Zealand became an opportunity for both Symbiotics and American dairy farmers.

American dairy farmers now had an incentive to improve their colostrum collection and handling techniques. In 2004, the only FDA-certified facility exclusively dedicated to processing bovine colostrum was built in Phoenix, Arizona and headed up by Dr. Keech. The stringent colostrum collection and processing standards for human consumption I helped establish were employed in this state-of-the-art facility. Even though it may seem like a no-brainer today, two decades ago, these gold standards of colostrum supplement manufacturing were considered nearly unheard of. Up until only recently, the dairy cows supplying colostrum were limited to those living and grazing in the Southwestern U.S. (Arizona, California, New Mexico). Due to increased worldwide demand for colostrum supplements, cows from Midwestern states have been brought online.

The advantage of sourcing colostrum from cows in the Southwest is that calving is not limited to just the spring season, as it is in New Zealand and other parts of the world. The mild temperatures of the Southwest allow for year-round birthing, so colostrum can be collected and processed throughout the year. This also has the advantage of ensuring the colostrum contains the most relevant ("freshest") antibodies for currently-circulating pathogens.

The accepted measure of colostrum quality and effectiveness is its immunoglobulin G (IgG) content. Since colostrum processing can affect both IgG levels and bioavailability, pasteurization time and temperature are critical to preserving IgG activity. Batch pasteurization, which is used in commercial milk production, can destroy upwards of half of the IgG; ultra high temperature (UHT) processing destroys all IgG activity along with most other proteins in colostrum. As the pasteurization temperature increases, the less time it takes to destroy the IgG. So, in addition to using flash pasteurization, assessing IgG levels with high-performance liquid chromatography (HPLC) throughout

---

Guidelines for Colostrum Sourcing & Processing

- Colostrum is sourced from the first milking of Grade A dairy cows that are certified healthy.
- Cows are pasture-fed or pasture-raised (as close to organic as possible).
- Cows are not supplemented with rBST (synthetic growth hormone).
- Cows are not routinely fed antibiotics.
- Colostrum is minimally processed to preserve the immune bioactives, growth factors, and other components.
- Colostrum is defatted to prevent rancidity.
- Lactose may be removed to lessen the allergic-like response of lactose intolerance.
- Liposomal Delivery coating is applied to increase bioavailability and ensure consistent solubility.
- Colostrum is processed according to Good Manufacturing Processes (GMP).
- End-product colostrum supplements undergo rigorous testing for safety and efficacy, including microbial analysis.
- Minimum IgG content of end-product colostrum supplement is 25%.

---

the manufacturing process is paramount. The range of IgG in properly processed colostrum is between 25-48% of the total protein content, with 25-30% IgG being ideal. Dr. Keech's facility was designed to consistently achieve these levels.

Dr. Keech is world renown for his proprietary colostrum peptide extraction techniques and expertise in the use of proline-rich polypeptides (PRPs) to regulate the immune system and stimulate the production of natural killer (NK) cells. His pioneering work with colostrum and colostrum-derived PRPs in HIV/AIDS patients is the quintessential application of peptide immunotherapy. An oral PRP spray developed and patented by Dr. Keech was studied in Phase I and Phase II clinical trials at the Infectious Disease Clinic in Dayton, Ohio (1996) and at the University of Nairobi in Nairobi, Kenya (2000), respectively and with promising results. Patients' CD4+ T-cells increased, viral load decreased, HIV/AIDS related physical symptoms resolved, and patients regained weight during the course of the study.[74] NK cells helped locate and destroy HIV-infected cells, thus identifying PRPs as the first viable immune-modulating natural substance in HIV/AIDS therapy.

My journey would not be complete without mention of another very special Kiwi – Graeme Clegg, the CEO of New Image Group, a business colleague, and a treasured friend. New Image Group is a New Zealand-based health and nutritional product provider and one of the oldest direct sales companies in the Asia-Pacific region. Because Graeme sells products that contain colostrum, we shared many of the same business contacts in New Zealand. Nearly two decades ago when we were mere acquaintances, Graeme became aware of a secretive takeover plot of Symbiotics. He alerted me, and I was able to stave off the takeover. We've been good friends ever since.

Previously, I mentioned the peaks and valleys in the colostrum industry. So, too have there been peaks and valleys in the part of my career involving colostrum…good characters, bad characters…but on the whole, I consider myself quite fortunate to have crossed paths with a lot of decent people. And of course, I had Kaye to support and nurture me along the way. She was the reason, after all, why I got into this business in the first place.

Furthermore, I still have faith that New Zealand can return to its original way of drying colostrum with low heat. New Zealand, with its pristine pasturelands, has the potential to once again produce the highest quality colostrum in the world.

6

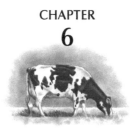

Is Your Gut Slowly Killing You?

Hippocrates was spot on when he said that all disease begins in the gut – just ask someone who suffers with IBS, Crohn's disease, or something as "mild" as occasional constipation or acid reflux. The thirty feet from mouth to anus that comprises the human G.I. tract represents a lot of real estate, of which any point along the way may be subject to injury. But for as debilitating as some well-known bowel conditions can be, there are hundreds of chronic diseases linked to gut health, and their prevalence has steadily risen in the last fifty years or so. Modern medicine has more recently begun to understand and accept the concepts of immune and gastrointestinal health as being intertwined and interdependent. Many chronic and autoimmune conditions stem from increased intestinal permeability and imbalances within the gut microbiome. If he were alive today, Hippocrates would likely assert that, *"All disease begins in a leaky gut."*

Presently, in 2020, the concept of *leaky gut, or leaky gut syndrome*, has been relegated to the practice of alternative medicine, and is only more widely accepted as a "real" condition by naturopaths (N.D.) and doctors of osteopathic medicine (D.O.); conventional medical doctors (M.D.) are less accepting and many deny or debate its existence. But this view is changing, and I believe the reason for the change is two-fold. First, we are learning more, as is always the case with better research methods and advances in technology. Second, more people are suffering from chronic and autoimmune diseases that were relatively uncommon in our not-so-distant past. This reality necessitates that we find out what the heck is going on so we can try to fix it. Otherwise, if we don't fix it, the personal and economic costs will be far greater than they already are, which is staggering to say the least.

The conventional medicine term for leaky gut is increased intestinal permeability. As a side note, the Wikipedia page for leaky gut syndrome (LGS) clearly points viewers in the direction of intestinal permeability.

This article is about a proposed medical condition in alternative medicine. For the phenomenon whereby the intestine wall exhibits excessive permeability, see Intestinal permeability.[75,76]

Wikipedia also refers to LGS as a pseudomedical diagnosis. I point this out not merely because not everything you read online is accurate, but I anticipate future updates as our collective medical knowledge and understanding of the relationship between human physiology and disease changes. After all, it wasn't all that long ago that Australian physician Barry Marshall and Australian pathologist Robin Warren were ridiculed for suggesting that *Helicobacter pylori* caused most peptic ulcers, rather than stress, spicy foods, and excessive stomach acid, as had been the belief for many decades at the time. On October 3, 2005, the duo was awarded the Nobel Prize in Medicine for proving that the *H. pylori* bacterium is the infectious cause of stomach ulcers. The story of *H. pylori* doesn't end there, so I ask you to put it on the proverbial back-burner in your mind. I'll return to it in the next chapter.

The term intestinal permeability broadly describes the control of substances in the G.I. tract passing into the bloodstream through the lining of the small intestine (i.e., the gut wall). This normal occurrence allows vitamins, minerals, electrolytes, and other nutrients from digested food to be absorbed by the body. In this respect, intestinal permeability is vital to our survival, but increased or excessive permeability is a health concern. The lining is comprised of epithelial ("skin") cells which normally form tight junctions, yet when these junctions loosen, there is increased permeability. If the gut wall is too permeable (i.e., junctions are too loose), potentially harmful substances such as undigested food proteins, antigens, microbial pathogens, and chemical toxins can also pass though the gut wall and thereby circulate to other parts of the body. Once in the bloodstream, the foreign materials attract the attention of the immune system which then mounts an inflammatory response to destroy and eliminate that which should not be in the bloodstream.

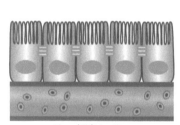
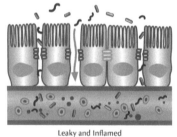

Normal Tight Junction   Leaky and Inflamed

Figure 3: Normal G.I. Lining vs. Increased Intestinal Permeability

When I speak to lay audiences, I find it helpful to paint a picture in people's minds about why increased intestinal permeability presents a significant threat to health and immune resiliency. I tell them to think of their intestines like sewer pipes, which carry the waste material from food digestion (i.e., feces) and from other contaminants consumed, either on foods or in water (i.e., pesticides, herbicides, environmental contaminants, bacteria, fungi, parasites). In a healthy gut, the sewer pipes are sturdy and without any holes, so the sewage goes about its business through the G.I. tract until you do your business in the toilet (a bowel movement). Conversely, if you have leaky sewer pipes, sewage seeps through the small holes and into the bloodstream where first, it doesn't belong and second, it can do damage.

So, although "increased intestinal permeability" may sound nice, "leaky gut" or "leaky gut syndrome" makes it infinitely more clear why this condition is so concerning. Chronically leaking pipes may spring bigger leaks and more leaks along the sewer line until you've got a great big mess! If a sewer pipe bursts in your home, there's usually a lot of damage and you need to call a plumber. Hopefully it's not on the weekend when overtime rates apply. Henceforward, I'll refer to the condition as leaky gut, lest that vivid image be forgotten.

One could argue a gut that leaks temporarily, as what is observed following high intensity or prolonged exercise, is okay as long as it doesn't become a pervasive problem. However, high caliber athletes as well as otherwise healthy individuals who experience leaky gut on an ongoing basis have an increased risk of the conditions associated with chronic inflammation. The beauty of the immune system is that in most people, it's extremely efficient. If some foreign material enters the bloodstream through the porous gut lining, the immune system detects and recognizes that this "invader" does not belong there. Then, it sends its "guards" to apprehend and remove the invader via an up-regulation of the inflammatory process. Once the invader is destroyed and inflammation is no longer necessary, the immune system down-regulates itself, inflammation subsides, and homeostasis returns.

Yet, if leaky gut becomes chronic, integrity of the G.I. lining is increasingly compromised. Inflammation also becomes chronic and instead of the immune system returning to a state of homeostasis, it too becomes a victim of chronic up-regulation. It begins to malfunction and mistake friend for foe, attacking healthy cells, healthy tissues, and healthy organs – not just the undigested food proteins, antigens, microbial pathogens, and chemical toxins. Once leaky gut becomes a vicious cycle – I call it leaky gut syndrome – the immune system creates antibodies against its own cells; this is autoimmunity. If left unabated, there is a tipping point at which recovery is improbable, and autoimmune diseases, such as rheumatoid arthritis, inflammatory bowel disease, type 1 diabetes, chronic fatigue syndrome, fibromyalgia, lupus, multiple sclerosis, psoriasis, scleroderma, thyroid diseases, vasculitis, and some mental health and neurocognitive disorders develop.

There are at least one-hundred officially recognized autoimmune diseases, and possibly many more unrecognized ones, categorized into two basic types – systemic and organ-specific. Systemic autoimmune diseases, such as rheumatoid arthritis, lupus, and scleroderma, affect multiple tissues and organs. Organ-specific autoimmune diseases affect one particular organ, such as type 1 diabetes (beta cells in the pancreas) or Graves' disease (thyroid). In general, the development of a specific autoimmune disease is related to the predominant location of the inflammation. For example, joint inflammation leads to rheumatoid arthritis, and gum inflammation leads to periodontal disease. Other factors, including aging, chronic stress, hormones, and pregnancy may compound the effects of a leaky gut and contribute to autoimmune diseases.

Inflammation in the gut itself also has consequences. It damages immunoglobulin A (IgA) whose job it is to protect the gut against pathogens. If IgA cannot neutralize the pathogens and the G.I. lining is abnormally permeable, the pathogens will enter the bloodstream, circulate, and infect other parts of the body. In response, the immune system increases its inflammatory response to deal with the pathogens, contributing to a vicious cycle of cellular havoc. The "syndrome" part of leaky gut syndrome (LGS) is a collection of symptoms which often pre-date – sometimes years or decades – a physician's diagnosis of an autoimmune disease. At first, these symptoms may present in the gut, such as heartburn, GERD, gas, bloating, constipation, and diarrhea, and although annoying or uncomfortable, most people reach for an over-the-counter (OTC) product to treat them. Now that so many previously prescription-only G.I. medications are available without a prescription, consumers are not only open to self-diagnosis, but to self-treatment without a second thought. We've been conditioned to believe that if a drug is available OTC, then it must be safe to use. Reliance and continued use of such products can in fact worsen leaky gut by damaging the delicate intestinal lining. More to come on the scourge of pharmaceuticals in the next chapter.

Food allergies are also a common symptom of LGS – something you'd probably not expect – yet, if you take a closer look, it makes perfect sense. When undigested food proteins, for example, from a beef patty or hamburger bun you just ate cross over into the bloodstream and trigger an inflammatory, or allergic reaction, by the immune system, that is considered a food allergy. As leaky gut worsens, the number of food allergies often increases, and sufferers find themselves with fewer and fewer non-allergenic food choices available to them. For many, the inability to eat the foods they once enjoyed gets into life satisfaction issues and may contribute to nutritional deficiencies in extreme cases. Many years ago, a woman told me that as time went on, the only food she could consume without problems was alligator meat – no joking.

The contributors to irritation of G.I. tissue and LGS are often self-inflicted, but generally unintentional. This is perhaps due, in part, to the lack of focus on LGS in conventional medicine, but it is important nonetheless and as LGS goes mainstream, the tide will surely change – I hope. Otherwise, we may realize too late that "death begins in the gut." Lifestyle and environmental antagonists possess varying degrees of influence, such that we can make many, some, or no changes in order to decrease the risk of LGS and autoimmune diseases. Those related to personal health behaviors (i.e., smoking, unhealthy eating) – we have lots of influence over. Those related to socio-economic or geographical situations (i.e., polluted air, food deserts) – we have much less influence over. The goal then, is to change or modify what we can and be aware of what we cannot.

Lifestyle Antagonists	Environmental Antagonists
oral antibiotics	antibiotics in food or water
NSAIDs/pain medications	glyphosate in food and water
corticosteroids	polluted air
hormonal birth control	contaminated drinking water
high sugar diet	contaminated soil
highly processed foods	parasites, pesticides
chemical food additives	GMO foods
gluten (for sensitive people)	yeast, and molds
excessive alcohol consumption	acid rain
excessive caffeine intake	wastewater, stormwater
smoking	lead, asbestos, dioxin

Hypotheses of leaky gut, or altered intestinal permeability as it was originally termed, and its connection to autoimmune diseases began emerging in the late 1980s. Two investigators, Kent Katz, M.D. and Daniel Hollander, M.D., gave perhaps one of the earliest mentions of leaky gut in their study of rheumatoid arthritis in 1989.[77] It reads in part:

Rheumatological disorders frequently have gastrointestinal manifestations and, conversely, intestinal disorders frequently have rheumatological manifestations. The possibility of altered intestinal permeability in arthritic patients may provide the bridge needed to link the two organ systems. The normal intestine absorbs nutrients and excludes the remaining material. If the intestine were less discriminating or 'leaky' then material normally excluded would be able to cross the intestinal mucosa into the lamina propria. An inflammatory response to these antigens, be they dietary, bacterial, or viral in origin, could produce either local or systemic disease. This would depend upon the type of immunological response and the cross-reactivity between the host's antigens and the absorbed antigens. This theory could account for the postulated relationship between intestinal abnormalities and the pathogenesis of some forms of arthritis.

In the last thirty years, as we learned more about leaky gut and its connection to the development of autoimmune diseases, we also learned how to measure it. Quantifying intestinal permeability does more than prove its existence, but measures it in relation to specific diseases and evaluates dietary or behavioral strategies – ones that can alter for good (health-promoting) or for bad (health-compromising). An early measure of intestinal permeability, which is still employed today because of its affordability and ease of use, is lactulose/mannitol urine testing. A baseline urine sample is obtained, followed by ingestion of a liquid solution comprised of two small sugar molecules (lactulose and mannitol), and a second urine sample is obtained after six hours; a comparison of pre- and post-amounts of lactulose and mannitol in the urine is correlated with intestinal permeability. The primary drawbacks of this test are that it is not truly reflective of larger food proteins that cross the gut lining nor do the two sugars themselves produce an immune reaction.

Another frequently used low-cost test is the Food Sensitivities Test. This at-home test measures the IgG reactivity levels (i.e., the immune reaction) in a small blood sample obtained from a finger prick. Test manufacturers compare the IgG reactivity to about one-hundred commonly consumed foods and provide a ranked list of foods to avoid. The Food Sensitivities Test does not require a doctor's prescription and is available to purchase on the Internet. As such, its primary function is consumer use – to suggest which foods will trigger an immune reaction. Eliminating these foods from one's diet may ease or eliminate symptoms, yet it does not fix the underlying problem of a leaky gut.

A more useful measure of intestinal permeability and one that is currently employed in clinical research is the Zonulin Test. Discovered in 2000 by Alessio Fasano, M.D. and colleagues at the University of Maryland School of Medicine, zonulin is a protein that modulates the degree of permeability between the cells that comprise the G.I. lining and its tight junctions.[78] Elevated zonulin levels indicate increased intestinal permeability. The Zonulin Test requires a blood draw by a physician or a stool sample, and results are most meaningful when utilized as part of a strategic plan to reduce the lifestyle antagonists that contribute to leaky gut.

As I mentioned earlier, food allergies are a symptom of LGS. Over the years, my contention has always been that you really don't need to take a commercially-available intestinal permeability test if you are experiencing food allergies or sensitivities. These tests may be helpful as a means of confirmation for either you or your physician and may serve as validation for any dietary changes you make (i.e., pre- and post-testing). In other words, it may be a nice thing to know, but you should skip the expense, which for many people, is not reimbursed by insurance. Instead, if you can heal your leaky gut, symptoms will subside and you'll feel better. There's no better validation than when your gut – and the rest of you – feels good.

In the last decade, we've turned our attention to the gut

microbiome, the ecosystem of trillions of microorganisms – bacteria, bacteria, viruses, and fungi – that call the thirty feet of G.I. real estate "home." The gut microbiome, affectionately referred to as our "gut bugs," regulates metabolism, manufactures vitamins and neurotransmitters, turns genes on and off, and communicates with other cells in the body. It is in fact, considered an organ itself, the so-called "second brain" which holds its own nervous system and communicates bi-directionally with the brain residing in the skull. The "telephone cord" from the gut microbiome to the brain is the vagus nerve, and it's the rationale behind the old saying, *I've got a gut feeling*.

The gut microbiome contains mostly good, or beneficial microorganisms, with the majority being bacteria, but some fungi species and viruses as well. There are also some bad, or pathogenic microorganisms cohabitating, but the good gut bugs generally keep the bad ones in check. This balance, or state of homeostasis is vital to immune health, since at least two-thirds of immune function resides in the gut. The microbiome plays a substantial role in modulating the immune system, whether it's promoting health or hindering it, so we must look to the "health" of the ecosystem. If the normal microbial balance is thrown out of whack for some reason (i.e., the bad gut bugs colonize beyond acceptable levels), there can be acute health consequences such as food poisoning (gastroenteritis) or the occasional cold or flu. Infections that are more chronic in nature include small intestinal bacterial overgrowth (SIBO), *candidiasis, Clostridium difficile*, and some urinary tract infections. The state of unbalanced gut bacteria is referred to as *dysbiosis*. A leaky gut compounds the problem of dysbiosis when these pathogenic microbes gain access to the bloodstream, which can have a deadly outcome – sepsis. Of the 1.7 million American adults who develop sepsis annually, nearly 270,000 will die.[79]

Remember: A non-permeable gut lining plus a healthy microbiome, allows many pathogenic microbes either be neutralized quickly or to pass out of the body in a bowel movement without ever gaining a foothold in the G.I. tract.

When the gut bugs are healthy, happy, and in balance, they share their happiness with the brain, and you experience this as positive mood. On the other hand, when they're unhealthy and unbalanced, your brain feels it too – as depression, bipolar disorder, and other mental illnesses. This is because healthy gut bacteria produce the brain's "feel good" chemicals – serotonin and dopamine – which travel up the vagus nerve to the brain. An ample supply of healthy bacteria is ideal since upwards of 90% of serotonin is produced in the gut. That's huge when you really think about it! Thus, keeping the gut microbiome healthy facilitates good mental health as well as physiological functioning within the entire body. This means actively managing your daily stress, eating a nutritious and clean diet, exercising regularly, getting plenty of quality sleep, and avoiding the various insults that compromise the microbiome. I'll talk more about antibiotics and pain medications in the next chapter, as these are two of the most prevalent and dangerous insults to gut health.

Let's back up for a moment so I can describe Dr. Fasano's contribution to our ever-increasing understanding about leaky gut and autoimmune diseases. He is of course, well known for characterizing leaky gut with the popular Las Vegas motto, *"Your gut is not like Vegas. What happens in the gut doesn't stay in the gut."* When Dr. Fasano and colleagues discovered zonulin and its connection to tight junction dysfunction, they gave us a new theory of how autoimmune diseases could develop in genetically susceptible patients;[80] when zonulin is up-regulated, the tight junctions become less tight, which ultimately leads to an elevated inflammatory response as antigens (i.e., undigested food proteins,

Inflammatory Diseases & Conditions Linked with Zonulin	
Celiac Disease	Asthma
Type 1 Diabetes	Coronary Artery Disease
Type 2 Diabetes	Irritable Bowel Syndrome
Inflammatory Bowel Disease	Non-Celiac Gluten Sensitivity
Ulcerative Colitis	Environmental Enteropathy
Multiple Sclerosis	Necrotizing Enterocolitis
Insulin Resistance	Septicemia (sepsis)
Obesity	Glioma
	Polycystic Ovary Syndrome

microbial toxins) from a dysbiotic gut are released into the bloodstream. This is, of course, an oversimplified explanation of Dr. Fasano's research, but it does provide a strong link between seemingly unrelated diseases – inflammation.

Dr. Fasano's follow-up research identified enteric (intestinal) bacteria which produce toxins, and gliadin, a protein in the gluten part of wheat, as the two primary triggers of zonulin release.[81] When this occurs in genetically-susceptible people, elevated zonulin then triggers a release of pro-inflammatory cytokines which in turn, activates T-cells of the immune system. The T-cells can do their damage by one of two pathways – stay in the G.I. tract or migrate to other organs – depending upon a person's genetic make-up. T-cells in the G.I. tract cause chronic inflammation in the gut, which leads to celiac disease and irritable bowel disease. A migration of T-cells outside the G.I. tract causes systemic inflammation and tissue damage, resulting in any number of autoimmune diseases, metabolic disorders, heart and lung diseases, and neurological diseases.

Dr. Fasano's research provides a glimmer of hope as well. His theory surrounding the up/down regulation of zonulin implies that once an autoimmunity process has begun, it doesn't necessarily have to be the perpetual outcome. In other words, by down-regulating zonulin, the intestinal lining function can return to normal (i.e., not leaky), and this would be a potential way to manage or potentially reverse autoimmune and chronic inflammatory diseases. Additionally, improving the health of the microbiome is critical. By keeping the pathogenic microbes at bay, even a temporary increase in intestinal permeability could theoretically limit the amount of toxic leakage and ensuing inflammatory damage.

So, again, I return to the importance of colostrum, as it relates to microbiome health and maintaining the integrity of the tight junctions to avoid leaky gut. First, various bioactives in colostrum, such as the oligosaccharides function as prebiotics to help support the growth and colonization of beneficial gut bacteria. Others, such as lactoferrin, lysozyme, lactoperoxidase and the immunoglobulins trigger the destruction of pathogenic bacteria. Second, epithelial growth factor and transforming growth factor-α help repair and restore integrity of the G.I. lining after zonulin is downregulated.

A 2017 study by a Polish research team lead by Maciej Hałasa, M.D., Ph.D. found that bovine colostrum supplementation reduced stool zonulin levels in athletes who were susceptible to increased intestinal permeability caused by vigorous exercise.[82] Iranian researchers examining intestinal permeability in ICU patients found that zonulin levels decreased when patients received bovine colostrum via enteral (tube) feeding.[83] This 2019 study also found that patients' endotoxin levels (toxins inside bacterial cells which are released when the cell disintegrates) significantly decreased by the 10th day of colostrum supplementation. These two studies show the diversity of bovine colostrum's application – from healthy athletes to critically ill patients.

We often speculate and hypothesize until we can design scientific studies that prove our theories, and double-blind, placebo-controlled human studies are the gold standard.

Yet, observational studies with human subjects are nothing to be sneezed at. What I'm trying to convey is that if a specific behavior (i.e., taking colostrum daily) produces a visible result, the mechanism (the "how") is less important than the actual result. That was certainly the case with Kaye as she steadily regained her health. After about a decade of taking colostrum, Kay and I took a food allergy / sensitivity test through Rocky Mountain Analytical (RMA) to satisfy our curiosity about measuring colostrum's effectiveness outside of our subjective experiences. Of the 187,000 tests that had been performed to date by RMA, only mine and Kaye's came back negative. Needless to say, the lab was very interested in what we were doing differently, and we were convinced of colostrum's health-enhancing action.

In the future, we will know more than we know today. Dr. Hałasa's research utilized knowledge from both Dr. Playford's studies that colostrum reduced leaky gut caused by heavy exercise and Dr. Fasano's discovery of zonulin as a regulatory and measurement of leaky gut. But in the meantime, I continue to advocate colostrum for everyone – whether you currently have an autoimmune disease or not. Many experts agree that we'll all die of an autoimmune disease – one that may take decades to fully develop. Yet, as it is developing – while leaky gut is happening – colostrum is our best "medicine" for healing the gut. Unless a permeable gut is healed, the body cannot begin to repair the damage caused by chronic inflammation. As healing begins, the quantity of antigens and toxins dumped into the bloodstream will decline and a cascade of positive outcomes will follow. Nutritional uptake will improve, and the cells will have better access to the fuel they need to for repair and regeneration; organ function will improve, energy levels will rise; immune resilience will return; and the greater sense of well-being will help us be the best version of ourselves.

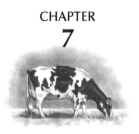

Microbiome Killers:
Scourge of the Pharmaceutical Industry

Hippocrates was a pillar of wisdom in the ancient world. His teachings sustained their relevancy over the centuries, and are perhaps even more relevant today. Hippocrates emphasized the importance of allowing the body to heal itself naturally with lifestyle and nutrition (i.e., wheatgrass, sprouts, edible algae); the goal was to create or reestablish harmony between an individual and his/her natural and social environment – mind, body, and spirit – much like our modern-day concept of wellness or well-being.[84] Medicine was only used if self-healing was unsuccessful. Great advice, but I would argue that along the way, Western physicians got a little side-tracked, especially with the exponential growth of a greedy pharmaceutical industry.

The problem with many (most) prescription and over-the-counter (OTC) medications is that while they're intended to relieve a particular symptom or "fix" a problem, they often contribute to a secondary problem. If you listen to any one of the prolific television advertisements for drugs, the amount of time it takes to recite the potential side effects is quite often longer than the first part of the ad. Furthermore, there are drugs to "fix" the problems that result from the use of other medications. Two of the main culprits affecting the integrity of the G.I. lining and the health of the microbiome are pain medications and antibiotics – two common classes of drugs that nearly everyone has taken at some point in their lives.

I am not against "wonder drugs." They certainly have their place and time, especially in life-threatening circumstances (i.e., antibiotics for serious infections) or end-of-life situations (i.e., powerful pain killers for cancer). But consumers should be aware of when mediations are appropriate and when they're not, as well as the health consequences of long-term use, including physical dependence. Physicians also need to be aware of patient misuse or overuse and strive to offer viable alternatives to the notion that *there's a pill for every ill*. The better solution is getting to the root cause of the illness, and many times, that begins in the gut. But let's take a look at how some of today's most common medications are affecting the G.I. tract and the microbiome.

Pain medications – both prescription and OTC varieties – pose a danger to the delicate lining of the stomach and small intestine. Not only can they increase intestinal permeability, but can cause stomach ulcers and intestinal bleeding which in some patients, has led to death. There's a general perception that OTC non-steroidal anti-inflammatory drugs (NSAIDs) are harmless for treating mild to moderate pain, but that's a big misperception. In 2000, UK researchers estimated that about one in 1,200 patients who took NSAIDs regularly for at least two months died, compared to those who did not take NSAIDs; this accounted for approximately 2000 deaths of UK residents annually.[85] Package inserts warn of G.I. bleeding, but most people likely don't realize that intestinal bleeding is such a potentially serious side effect.

Furthermore, many people and healthcare practitioners are also just beginning to understand the implications of increased intestinal permeability, or leaky gut. A research review of conventional NSAID use showed that within twenty-four hours of ingestion, permeability increased.[86] An aspirin here and there for a headache or an occasional ibuprofen for muscle aches isn't going to kill anyone, but regular use, or dependence on prescription opioids is problematic. If you already have leaky gut caused by other lifestyle or environmental antagonists, the problem is compounded, so if you must use painkillers, especially opioids, use them for the least amount of time possible. And, lest we forget that regular NSAID use has other side effects, including increased risk of fatal and non-fatal heart attack, heart failure, stroke, elevated blood pressure, liver, and kidney problems.

The U.S. National Center for Health Statistics and National Center for Chronic Disease Prevention and Health Promotion collaborated on a survey of prescription opioid use among American adults and found that legal use increases as people grow older.[87] Between the years 2013 and 2016, 6.5% of Americans reported taking a prescription opioid in the previous thirty days – 3.2% of individuals aged 20 to 39; 7.5% of individuals aged 40 to 59; and 9.6% of individuals over sixty. Conservatively, twenty million American adults are taking a prescription opioid at any given time, plus the untold number of people using opioids illegally, and the sixty million NSAID users – and that's just one category of medication that contributes to leaky gut. So, I think you'll agree not only are there a lot of people in physical pain, but that the breath of leaky gut is quite wide within the U.S. population.

A 2012 epidemiological study reported that abdominal pain prompted more physician visits than any other G.I. symptom, and that G.I. diseases substantially contribute to illness, death, and cost in the U.S.[88] A 2018 update to this study determined that with more than 40.7 million visits for G.I. symptoms and 54.4 million visits for a diagnosed G.I. disease, the annual healthcare cost was $135.9 billion dollars.[89] Unfortunately, when patients go to their doctor seeking pain relief, they often receive a prescription for a steroid medication to reduce inflammation and pain, which simply exacerbates the destruction of G.I. tissue. Because physicians are more aware of opioid addiction today, they may recommend something with less addiction potential or even an OTC pain medication, but they're often in the dark about leaky gut. A prescription for any type of pain medication is essentially a prescription for leaky gut syndrome. And let's face it, consumers of medical services (a.k.a. patients) want what they want, and no one wants to suffer. That's completely understandable. *If I have pain and I go to my doctor, I want to leave with a solution – otherwise, I'll go elsewhere. My $20 co-pay requires something in return.*

And that brings me to another issue: Many physicians – while completely knowledgeable about medication side effects – don't want to jeopardize their patient relationships. So, whether it's not wanting valuable healthcare dollars to go elsewhere, or simply not wanting to further investigate a patient's pain, the script pad comes out and some type of pills are ultimately dispensed. The flawed rationale and flawed treatment of the past must be eliminated to faithfully fulfill the *do no harm* part of the Hippocratic oath. A better solution is for physicians to explain why pain medications are dangerous and instead, work with the patient to get to the root cause of the pain. This involves listening, patient education, and without a doubt, more of the physician's time.

Oral antibiotics are another class of medication that contributes to an unhealthy microbiome and in recent years, we've begun witnessing the consequences of the "nuclear bomb" approach to infectious bacteria. Prescribing broad-spectrum antibiotics indiscriminately creates more problems than it solves because in doing so, both good and bad gut bacteria are destroyed and some of the stronger, drug-resistant strains are left behind to colonize. Eventually, these become the dreaded "superbugs" for which there are fewer antibiotics capable of eradicating them. According to the CDC's 2019 report *Antibiotic Resistance in the United States*, more than 2.8 million antibiotic-resistant infections occur annually, and these infections kill more than 35,000 people.[90]

A single course of antibiotics can disrupt the normal balance of the microbiome, so just imagine what multiple courses will do. Even if the microbiome was able to recover to some extent on its own, it's continually playing catch-up, all the while contending with other extraneous factors affecting the microbiome (i.e., poor nutrition, too much stress, inadequate sleep). If an individual also has leaky gut, an overgrowth of bad gut-based bacteria and their toxins may seep into the bloodstream, and what was once limited to the G.I. tract, now becomes a systemic infection.

The majority of pathogens enter the human body through or attached to the mucosal surfaces, including the eyes, nose, and mouth. The nose and mouth provide access to the 30 feet of G.I. real estate, of which the small intestine is "prime property." Frequently, non-symptomatic people unwittingly share their gut bugs with others who have compromised immune systems. This is often the case with hospital-acquired infections (HAI) such as *Clostridioides dificile (C. diff.)* and methicillin resistant *Staphylococcus aureus* (MRSA). The gut bacteria get a free ride into the hospital or care facility with one person and go home with another person or multiple people. When an otherwise healthy carrier – with fecal matter on his or her hands – enters a hospital and touches any surface (i.e., handrail, elevator button, door, tray table, patient bed), the bacteria are transferred to that surface and the ones that survive can be picked up by another person (i.e., patient, visitor, nurse, doctor) and spread around. The final target of the bacteria is an immunocompromised patient who, in one way or another, absorbs the bacteria via his or her own mucosal surface(s), and voila!

The Centers for Disease Control and Prevention (CDC) estimates that one in thirty-one patients (3.2%) has an HAI on any given day while in the hospital.[91] In 2015, this accounted for 687,000 infections in acute care hospitals, of which approximately 72,000 patients died during their hospital stay. Due to increased surveillance and improved standards, these statistics are an improvement from 2011 when the same survey team estimated an HAI prevalence rate of 4%. This reduction corresponds to a 16% lower risk of developing an HAI, and while any improvement is good, it doesn't take into account the patients who are discharged with lurking infection – sicker than when they were initially admitted – and tragically die days, weeks, or months later. Those victims may never be counted.

Antibiotics are used for a wide range of bacterial infections and again, and I want to stress that this class of drugs is at times, essential and lifesaving, yet over-prescribing and incorrect prescribing are problematic both in the moment and long-term. Two very common situations which come to mind are urinary tract infections and seasonal flu. Urinary tract infections (UTIs) are the second most common infection and result in about 8.1 million doctor visits annually.[92] UTIs can sometimes go away on their own, but generally require antibiotics to prevent a more serious infection from spreading to the kidneys. The problem lies in the time it takes to culture a urine sample to determine which strain of bacteria is responsible for the infection. Meanwhile, the healthcare practitioner prescribes a broad-spectrum antibiotic to eliminate the infection which may or may not be the best choice. Furthermore, how many patients have phoned their doctor to describe UTI symptoms (because they've had UTIs in the past), and the doctor calls in a prescription to the pharmacy without ever culturing a urine specimen? What about recurring UTIs for which no attempt is made to ascertain and address the underlying cause? The ongoing decimation of the gut microbiome leads to other health problems and contributes to antibiotic resistance.

Prescribing antibiotics for the seasonal flu – or any viral infection for that matter – is absolutely absurd, but strangely, not unheard of. In 2013, the CDC's report Antibiotic Resistance Threats in the United States laid responsibility at the door of physicians who misuse antibiotics by either prescribing too many of them or by prescribing them inappropriately.[93] The CDC noted that up to 50% of the prescriptions written were not necessary or the dosage was incorrect. Unfortunately, it's often a case of a strong-willed patient who bullies a healthcare provider into writing a script for something that has no effect on viruses. Physicians know better, but often give in, lest they lose a customer and the patient moves on to someone more willing to cater to their demands. That's what I find so maddening, and I encourage physicians to be stern and spend a little extra time and effort – perhaps, lots of effort – to educate patients why taking an antibiotic for a viral infection is misguided as well as dangerous to their health. So, physicians: it's perfectly okay to say "no," and let the patient's own immune system fight the virus. Otherwise, you are complicit in drug dealing of microbiome killers.

Fortunately, the concept of *antibiotic stewardship* is gaining traction worldwide. Physicians and other health professionals are gravitating towards the principles of responsible antibiotic prescribing. By curtailing indiscriminate use, the likelihood of antibiotics being effective in the future increases, and this is extremely important now that fewer new antibiotics are coming to market. No one wants to face the nightmare scenario of a raging bacterial infection for which absolutely no effective treatment is available. The good news is that antibiotics stewardship appears to be working. The CDC's 2019 report describes 18% fewer deaths and 28% fewer HAI related deaths from antibiotic resistance since their 2013 report. Vigilance and proactive measures remain critical to immune resilience because a lot of bad bugs are still out there, and the emergence of SARS-CoV-19 reminds us that viral threats are very much still in play.

Urgent Threats
- Carbapenem-resistant *Acinetobacter*
- *Candida auris*
- *Clostridioides difficile*
- Carbapenem-resistant *Enterobacteriaceae*
- Drug-resistant *Neisseria gonorrhoeae*

Serious Threats
- Drug-resistant *Campylobacter*
- Drug-resistant *Candida*
- ESBL-producing *Enterobacteriaceae*
- Vancomycin-resistant *Enterococci*
- Multidrug-resistant *Pseudomonas aeruginosa*
- Drug-resistant nontyphoidal *Salmonella*
- Drug-resistant *Salmonella serotype Typhi*
- Drug-resistant *Shigella*
- Methicillin-resistant *Staphylococcus aureus*
- Drug-resistant *Streptococcus pneumoniae*
- Drug-resistant Tuberculosis

Concerning Threats
- Erythromycin-resistant group A *Streptococcus*
- Clindamycin-resistant group B *Streptococcus*

Watch List
- Azole-resistant *Aspergillus fumigatus*
- Drug-resistant *Mycoplasma genitalium*
- Drug-resistant *Bordetella pertussis*

Patients: you aren't off the hook either because you most certainly are a stakeholder in your own health. (In Chapter 11, I'll discuss the concept of health sovereignty.) Any non-medically inclined person who has reached this far and still believes antibiotics are completely safe and without side effects, I encourage you to read the medical horror story of Mark Ghalili, D.O., a Los Angeles doctor who took a commonly-prescribed antibiotic and experienced debilitating health effects that left him paralyzed. Dr. Ghalili shares his story of Cipro toxicity (antibiotic poisoning) at the end of this chapter.

Even if you are a stellar example of immune resilience and never need to take antibiotics, you are still likely to consume antibiotic residues if you eat conventionally-raised meat, poultry, or fish. Most large livestock operations routinely feed antibiotics to cattle, pigs, and chicken, even in the absence of illness, and in the U.S., nearly 80% of oral antibiotics sold are utilized in livestock feed. The misguided, profit-driven goal is to fend off potential infections that can easily spread among animals living in tight quarters and to promote quicker (and unnatural) muscle tissue growth. This practice helps create strains of antibiotic-resistant bacteria, which when humans encounter, are impervious to our drugs.

Conventionally-raised beef is more likely to test positive for antibiotic-resistant bacteria such as *E. coli* and MRSA, and an interesting 2013 study found evidence pointing to high-density, factory-scale hog facilities as a source of MRSA in surrounding communities.[94] People living near hog farms or in areas where hog manure is applied to crops as fertilizer have an increased risk of contracting MRSA. People with the highest exposure to manure, based on how close they lived to farms, farm acreage, and quantity of manure used, were 38% more likely to get MRSA than the lowest exposure level.

My experience with hog farmers in the early 2000s, along with Michail Borissenko, M.S. at the Institute of Colostrum Research convinced me that antibiotics should never be routinely administered to promote growth in meat animals. Mr. Borissenko's research showed that newborn piglets benefitted more if they were fed bovine colostrum instead of the standard chow plus antibiotics.[95,96] Piglet mortality rate was lower, and the piglets matured quicker and were healthier overall. As a bonus, their meat was leaner, which inadvertently helped fulfill the pork industry's promotion of pork as "the other white meat." The farmers benefitted because they could bring the adult hogs to market sooner with less cost, which of course, translates to higher profits. The only rational (and conscionable) reason to give animals antibiotics is if they are sick, and any animal identified as such should be isolated from the others to prevent infection spread.

Most of us would agree that giving meat animals – cows, hogs, goats, chickens, turkeys, and even fish – unnecessary antibiotics hurts people in the long-term, and some farmers have voluntarily committed to reducing the amount they administer. The FDA's Center for Veterinary Medicine (CVM) has been phasing in a 2017 law which requires a vet's prescription, or a veterinary feed directive (VFD), for antibiotics administered in feed and water; prior to this, animal producers could purchase antibiotics from their local feed store or online. On the surface, this seems like a step in the right direction, yet it still means that a sick animal will receive antibiotic treatment if a VFD is issued.

Crowded animal living conditions – versus open pastures – are simply more likely to incubate and spread infections which necessitate VFDs. And so, when you're in the grocery store, do you have visions of thousands of chickens clucking shoulder-to-shoulder in a huge warehouse-like building? How do you really know what that chicken (or cow or pig) was fed with – even if it was raised according to all applicable laws? On a positive note, the FDA's CVM is committed to support antimicrobial stewardship in food-producing animals because they understand the seriousness of not taking action.[97]

Depending on your drinking water supply, you may also ingest antibiotic residues from farm run-off (animal waste) and manure-based fertilizers that have been applied to food crops. Furthermore, our own effluent – every time we flush the toilet or use primitive facilities – well, that contamination must eventually wind up somewhere. Residues from antibiotics, antidepressants, antihypertensives, hormonal contraceptives, and pain medications often end up in downstream water which feeds local municipalities.[98] So, unless you're living high on a mountaintop with clean food and water and pristine air, it's fair to say that human consumption of medication residues and other chemical toxins is unavoidable.

You can reduce your exposure to antibiotic residues by selecting pasture-raised meats and poultry from your local farmer's market or community supported agriculture (CSA) group. These animals are generally healthy, do not require antibiotics, and develop naturally in unconfined spaces. Due to the growing consumer demand for less antibiotics in meat and poultry products, many grocery stores now offer products that are "raised without antibiotics." And don't forget: These recommendations apply to animal food products as well – milk, butter, cheese, and eggs.

Even when you're committed to healthier food choices, you still need to contend with cross-contamination, especially if you or a family member is immunocompromised. Store-bought raw chicken products are frequently contaminated with illness-causing bacteria, even those that are labelled "organic" or "raised without antibiotics." *Consumer Reports* infamous 2013 analysis of more than three-hundred store-bought raw chicken breasts revealed that 97% were contaminated. The most common bacteria detected was Enterococcus, which occurred in 79.8% percent of the samples, followed by *E. coli* (65.2%); campylobacter (43%); *klebsiella pneumonia* (13.6%); salmonella (10.8%); and *staphylococcus aureus* (9.2 %). Furthermore, nearly half (49.7%) of the samples tested contained at least one type of antibiotic-resistant bacteria, and another 11.5% contained two or more types of multidrug-resistant bacteria. Chicken is the most popular meat consumed in the U.S., and although consumers are advised to handle all raw meat carefully and cook it to the appropriate temperature, the CDC acknowledges more deaths attributable to poultry than to any other commodity.

Certainly, as we learn more about the foods we eat, medications we take, and environments in which we live, we can advocate for change and commit to making realistic changes in our own lives. The superbugs created by prior decades of antibiotic misuse and our over-reliance and addictions to pain medications need not be our undoing. That's where bovine colostrum has an important role to play, one that is exceedingly critical at this point in time. And unlike the so-called wonder drugs of the pharmaceutical industry, absolutely no harm comes from taking colostrum.

Unlike antibiotics manufactured in a laboratory, bovine antibodies are manufactured naturally in response to a female cow's exposure to various bacteria, viruses, and fungi she encounters while grazing in the pasture or coming in contact with her human caretakers.[99,100] When the colostrums from hundreds of cows are pooled together, the antibody diversity increases significantly – much to our own health advantage. We also get antimicrobial support from lactoferrin, lactoperoxidase, lysozyme, and proline-rich polypeptides in a multi-pronged approach towards minimizing or eliminating the need for pharmaceutical antibiotics.[101,102] Daily colostrum supplementation is essential to protecting the G.I. system from the occasional episode of food poisoning from the local eatery caused by *E. coli* to the life-threatening *C. diff* infection following a routine orthopedic surgery.

This leads to my general premise that a *balanced* gut microbiome is key to immune resilience and overall health...and for a remarkably simple reason. The "bad" microbes are unable to grow and reproduce themselves; they are held in-check by the "good" microbes. Yet, if the microbiome is unbalanced, the "bad" microbes can thrive and cause harm either to immune health or brain health (via the vagus nerve). Colostrum is important to the microbiome as it does two things: promotes the destruction of pathogenic microbes and promotes the growth of beneficial microbes.

Colostrum also helps maintain integrity of the tight junctions that comprise the intestinal lining. As I described in Chapter 5, the focus of Raymond Playford, M.D.'s early research was to investigate whether bovine colostrum could affect damaged G.I. tissue resulting from NSAID use. Dr. Playford and others have demonstrated that colostrum can indeed prevent NSAID-induced small intestine injury in both animal and human models.[103,104,105,106] This is certainly good news – although not necessarily a greenlight to use – for patients who take NSAIDs. A more integrous ("non-leaky") gut lining will prevent "foreign substances" from entering the bloodstream, creating an inflammatory response, and potentially contributing or causing more serious illnesses. Furthermore, the anti-inflammatory properties of colostrum may help reduce the need for NSAIDs and other pain medications in the first place – a basic, yet multifunctional supplement for living successfully in today's complicated world.

Doctor Battles Back Against Antibiotics
In 2016, board-certified internal medicine physician

Mark Ghalili, D.O. was prescribed a three-day course of Cipro – like many Americans – for a bacterial infection, and shortly afterwards, he began experiencing numerous progressive and debilitating symptoms. The muscle wasting, neuropathy, and seizures were so severe, that Dr. Ghalili found himself confined to a wheelchair – essentially paralyzed. He also experienced brain fog, severe anxiety, heart palpitations, and suicidal thoughts. Dr. Ghalili is living proof that Cipro toxicity is a real and very scary medical condition. If he hadn't experienced it himself, it may have been filed away under rare medication side effects, despite the increasing number of people suffering from similar, seemingly unrelated symptoms.

The initial signs that led Dr. Ghalili to believe he was ill were muscle weakness and tightness – common side effects of a simple workout. As an avid exerciser, Dr. Ghalili believed a light jog would help test his leg muscle capability, but mid-run, he found himself unable to move his legs, collapsed on the ground, and barley able to stand. He describes the pain as if a bomb went off in his body. Thankfully, he was able to find someone to take him home.

Cipro toxicity, the common reference to fluoroquinolone toxicity, has been associated with severe, wide-ranging side effects, including torn tendons, muscle pain and wasting, neurological conditions, depression, anxiety, psychosis, and suicidal ideation. Despite the FDA's 2016 warning that fluoroquinolone antibiotics (Cipro®, Levaquin®, Avelox®) should only be used to treat infections for which other antibiotics are ineffective, they are routinely prescribed for common infections – urinary tract infections, chronic bacterial prostatitis, chronic bronchitis, lower respiratory tract infections, sinusitis, and infectious diarrhea. For years, patients were cautioned about not exercising their Achilles tendon too strenuously after taking Cipro due to the risk of rupture and tendonitis, but that was the extent of it. In 2008, the FDA issued a warning about that specific risk because they had received reports of ruptured tendons in the shoulder and hand as well as the ankle.

It's likely that with such a wide range of side effects recognized today, patients (and many physicians) don't make the association right away, especially since symptoms may not appear for sixty to ninety days after taking Cipro. Even many of Dr. Ghalili's colleagues didn't believe it – or him! Fortunately, Dr. Ghalili lives and practices medicine in Los Angeles, so he had a bit of an advantage over other patients suffering with Cipro toxicity. His research showed that in lesser metropolitan areas, people were much more likely to be prescribed antibiotics in general and often unnecessarily – without a positive urine or other type of culture analysis.

When health issues arise, human nature is to ask why? and then to learn as much as possible, so just imagine what a physician-patient can learn. Dr. Ghalili's quest to heal himself has made him a leading expert in fluroquinolone toxicity, and his expertise will motivate you to avoid fluroquinolones like the plague. According to Dr. Ghalili's research, the metabolism (breakdown) of these antibiotics leads to an accumulation of free radicals that damages mitochondrial DNA, which in turn, leads to destruction of cells that comprise the musculoskeletal and central nervous systems. Fluroquinolone toxicity is cumulative so that the more antibiotics a patient takes over time, the greater the risk of oxidative stress and cell death affecting every organ in the human body – the brain, heart, lungs, kidneys, nervous system, musculoskeletal system, and connective tissue. The cellular changes to the mitochondria can disrupt energy production for years, and the genetic mutations are also long-lasting. Dr. Ghalili believes that fluroquinolone toxicity plays a role in both fibromyalgia and chronic fatigue syndrome.

In time, Dr. Ghalili was able to heal himself and no longer requires the use of a wheelchair. The journey was arduous, yet everything he learned along the way has enabled him to help patients with the same condition. He can honestly tell patients that he understands what they are experiencing, and since 2017, Dr. Ghalili has seen or treated more than 800 patients in his practice, Regenerative Medicine LA. With a focus on reestablishing mitochondrial health, restoring the gut microbiome, and rebuilding the immune system, his protocols utilize stem cell therapy, customized intravenous nutritional therapies, hormone therapy, a healthy diet, and bovine colostrum supplementation. As patients start to recover, and their bodies find homeostasis, the process of restoring muscular strength begins – with exercise and colostrum – which together are the foundations of athletic training and performance. To learn more about fluroquinolone toxicity and the wide array of regenerative treatments Dr. Ghalili offers, visit his website (regenerativemedicinela.com).

So long as I'm on the topic of the pharmaceutical industry, it's worth singling out Monsanto (acquired by Bayer in 2018) for its microbiome-destroying herbicide glyphosate, which is sold as Roundup®. In 1970, Monsanto chemist John E. Franz discovered this organophosphorus compound to be an effective, broad-spectrum weed killer and in 1974, it became available to farmers who wanted an easier way to eliminate the weeds and grasses that competed with their crops. Roundup® was also available at the local garden center or nursery for home use, so no more pulling of weeds by hand. Just a quick spritz of the desiccant, and weeds were dead the next day. As the decades went by, use of Roundup® skyrocketed; it was literally everywhere – on every farm and in every backyard garden.

Farmers may appreciate the weed-killing benefit of glyphosate for increased crop production, but probably few of them understand the lurking health dangers. In 2016, the World Health Organization's International Agency for Research on Cancer (IARC) labeled the glyphosate herbicide a "probable human carcinogen."[107] The IARC review committee made this determination based on their review of studies which found glyphosate in farmworkers' blood and urine, chromosomal damage in cells, and increased risk of non-Hodgkin lymphoma in some people who had been exposed; tumor formation in some animal studies has also been reported.

In recent years, Bayer has faced numerous lawsuits alleging that Roundup® causes cancer in humans and that's probably what you're most familiar with, but there's something even more ubiquitous and insidious. In the way that glyphosate kills weeds in the soil, it also kills the good bacteria ("weeds") in the G.I. tract. Studies in mice also show that glyphosate altered the normal microbial composition by reducing abundance and diversity; specifically, it led to a decrease in *Firmicutes, Bacteroidetes,* and *Lactobacillus,* which was then correlated with an increase in anxiety and depression-like behavior.[108] Research suggests links between glyphosate and antibiotic resistance and endocrine disruption.[109,110]

If glyphosate causes dysbiosis and an overgrowth of

pathogenic gut bacteria, then gut inflammation and leaky gut aren't far behind. I believe that glyphosate also destroys the villi in the gut, which in turn, reduces the absorbability of vitamins and minerals. The increased use of glyphosate since the mid-1970s appears to correlate with the spike in celiac disease and other autoimmune conditions. So much of the American diet is comprised of corn, wheat, and soy – prime targets for spraying of Roundup®. We are literally eating herbicides on a daily basis, so it's reasonable to make the connection to leaky gut. Furthermore, maternal exposure to glyphosate and other toxic chemicals is a concern for a developing fetus.

Glyphosate is the world's most widely-used herbicide with more than 160 countries applying 1.4 billion pounds of it annually. Just about every wheat, corn, soybean and cotton crop grown in the U.S. is sprayed with glyphosate. Data from California shows that in 2012 glyphosate was applied to five million acres of almonds, peaches, cherries, citrus, grapes, cantaloupes, onions, and other edible crops. Timing of glyphosate application is also consequential, and pre-harvest use results in very high residues.

The easiest solution, as you would think, is to go organic, or gluten, corn, and soy-free, but not so fast…it's complicated unnecessarily. When glyphosate is aerially sprayed, it often drifts to other crops, even ones that have not being treated with glyphosate. In other words, an organic farmer's tomato crop could become contaminated by virtue of a neighboring crop that has been sprayed. Or, if your organic milk comes from cows that have been grazing near a conventionally-sprayed cotton field, it may contain glyphosate residues. Glyphosate can also evaporate into the clouds, which then travel miles away and rain down on an unsuspecting organic farmer's crops.

I think you get the idea as to why glyphosate contamination has become ubiquitous in our food supply. Unfortunately, even foods that are grown organically yet subjected to glyphosate drift can still be labeled "organic." Testing the amount of glyphosate in food is not a common practice, but as more people sound the alarm, testing will be done in the hopes that one day, glyphosate will be banned in the United States as some countries have already done.

Reducing Your Toxic Exposure

- Eat organic whenever possible.
- Know where your food is grown or grow your own.
- Choose foods from local farmers markets or community sponsored agriculture programs.
- Thoroughly wash fresh fruits and vegetables.
- Avoid or minimize soy, corn, wheat and wheat-containing products.
- Consume grass-fed or pastured meats.
- Support farmers who do not use glyphosate.
- Get involved in the effort to ban glyphosate.

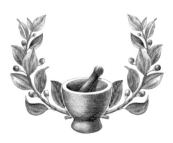

"

The most advanced, creative and original thinking is always a product if historical context and the influences of previous geniuses, mentors, and collaborators on the mind of the originator.

Michael J. Gelb

"

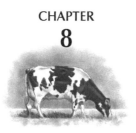

What Doctors Don't Know Can Harm You

Doctors are human – just like the rest of us. Yet for large chunk of human history, the medical profession was right up there with the clergy in terms of influence over daily life. Religion and medicine were so important to survival that individuals who held positions of authority in either arena, also wielded significant power within the community. In fact, there's an old Indian saying that describes doctors as being second to God on this earth (a.k.a. "the God complex"). Certainly, when Kaye and I were growing up and for many people of our generation, this was the case. Perhaps it can be attributed to a physician's power to save lives, as Voltaire described:

"Those who are occupied in the restoration of health to others, by the joint exertion of skill and humanity, are above all the great of the earth. They even partake of divinity, since to preserve and renew is almost as noble as to create."

Our religious faith played an influential role in our lives and that of our families, and although that aspect never wavered, our faith in doctors did. It became clear to us as the years went by, and as people shared their health stories with us, that modern doctors were failing their patients miserably. Well, maybe not intentionally, but when combined with no patient pushback on the God complex, doctors enjoyed misappropriated stature while many patients suffered needlessly.

There's also an element of *we know more today*. This helps avoid epic medical mistakes of the past, such as radiating children's thymus glands, but often old mistakes get replaced by new mistakes. Upon reflection, it's the more we know is the more we realize just how much we don't know. Fortunately, if we take that to heart, we'll never stop learning. Like Kaye's story and Dr. Mark Ghalili's story illustrate the life-changing impact of an accepted medical treatment, they also inspire us to take ownership of, be responsible for, and participate in our own health. And this is what I refer to as "health sovereignty."

The concept of health sovereignty emerged from my and Kaye's journey to rediscover colostrum as the elemental foundation of life – and immune health. Somewhere along the fast track to modernization, people forgot about colostrum. It was set aside when new technologies, new medications, and new vaccines became available. Why would anyone need colostrum beyond infancy (or at all) when there's a magnanimous pharmaceutical industry working tirelessly developing medications for every health problem known to us – and maybe even a few novel conditions inadvertently created from the side effects of said medications? Just think about that for a moment…and then think about this: What if the "secret" to health was the very gift your mother gave you the day you were born? Some may believe there's a spiritual meaning in this, and others may believe it to be simple biology, but whichever view you take, a growing number of health practitioners and health-minded people have taken notice.

In the past, it sometimes felt like Kaye and I were colostrum pariahs. Since neither of us had a medical background, we struggled to get the message to those who could actually recommend colostrum to patients. In fact, we frequently found ourselves pleading for patients to tell their doctors about colostrum and refer them back to us for more information. In the rare case that a doctor would actually call us to discuss colostrum, we were thrilled – because it meant educating one more person who could then make a difference for someone else. Occasionally, we'd stumble upon a doctor who tried colostrum for him or herself – usually an act of personal desperation – and experienced a positive outcome. We were immensely appreciative of anyone in the mainstream medical community who was willing to share their healing stories with us. Of course, this didn't always translate to them recommending it to their own patients. The old saying about doctors being the worst patients is probably true, but I have faith that they can also be some of the best self-health advocates when given the appropriate platform. Of course, this is so much easier in the age of the Internet and social media.

One of the "powers" afforded to physicians is that of discernment when it comes to prescribing or recommending therapies, and it's predicated on their extensive formal education and training in their respective medical fields. Essentially, it allows them to – in the course of treating their own patients – make health claims about various drugs, health products and/or therapies – something which the Food and Drug Administration (FDA) disallows for non-medically trained individuals (i.e., the rest of us). The FDA's (and also the FTC's) intent is to protect consumers from manufacturers' outrageous marketing claims about products that they might take or use in place of accepted, traditional medical treatment. The "outrageous" qualifier is debatable in my opinion, and I am certainly biased towards colostrum, but with good reason. After more than twenty-five years, I have seen its transformative effect on immune resilience – healing is more than just science. Although, the science is catching up.

What follows are a few brief stories from medical practitioners I asked to share their personal and professional
experiences with bovine colostrum.

Andrew BeDell, D.C.
Chiropractor on a Crusade

Missouri chiropractor Andrew BeDell, D.C. has quite a har-
rowing personal health story of gut health and cancer. In
the spring of 2015, Dr. BeDell was suddenly overcome with
bowel cramping and excruciating pain. His primary care
physician scheduled a colonoscopy, but that was one ap-
pointment Dr. BeDell would not be keeping. Instead, he
rushed to the E.R. and after a CT scan and blood work,
found himself undergoing emergency colostomy surgery –
the result of diverticulitis and a ruptured sigmoid colon.
After six months of healing and to great relief, Dr. BeDell's
surgeon reversed his colostomy.

Then, one day in the fall of 2017 while Dr. BeDell was
showering, he noticed the yellowing of his skin, the unmis-
takable sign of jaundice. He was later diagnosed with pancreatic cancer and underwent the Whipple procedure
(pancreaticoduodenectomy), a surgical procedure to remove
the cancerous tumor on the head of his pancreas. Two
weeks after surgery, Dr. BeDell had his first – and last – chemotherapy treatment. The side effects of chemotherapy gave
him pause to think about whether he could try a more
natural approach – something that wouldn't make him as
miserable and sick as "standard" treatment.

His first step was to eliminate all sugar from his diet, a
decision that many cancer patients opt to do. He also tried
various herbs and a thymus extract supplement to help
improve his immune system, but unfortunately, his health
challenges didn't end there. A self-diagnosis of small intestinal bacterial overgrowth (SIBO) combined with dull, flaky,
and silvery skin – perhaps dermatitis or psoriasis – was a

reflection of his poor gut health, and a PET scan revealed spots on his lungs. While Dr. BeDell mulled over having a lung biopsy, he came across an article about leaky gut and colostrum in a chiropractic journal. The notion of using nature's wisdom to return the body to a state of homeostasis so that it could heal itself made complete sense, so Dr. BeDell began supplementing his diet with bovine colostrum (2 Tbsp. 4 times/day) in the spring of 2018. The first thing Dr. BeDell noticed was the intense and frequent flatulence, which necessitated frequent apologies to his patients. But after two or three weeks as the SIBO came under control and the bad bacteria died off, the flatulence went away and his bowel health improved. After three months on colostrum, Dr. BeDell's energy levels had increased dramatically, so much so that he was inspired to join the local gym and hire a personal trainer.

By June, Dr. BeDell was feeling his old self again and went in for the dreaded lung biopsy. Much to the pulmonologist's amazement, there were no cancerous lesions. Dr. BeDell was equally amazed, but now he was facing a new crisis. A good friend of his was on the same trajectory – pancreatic cancer, followed by lung cancer – but went through standard chemotherapy and eventually died after great suffering. Dr. BeDell remembers his friend's wife lamenting as to why God took her husband and spared him. At times, survivor's guilt still haunts him. Yet, he is happy to be alive and well himself, knowing that he too could have suffered the same outcome.

In 2020, at age sixty-nine, Dr. BeDell advocates a naturopathic approach to health and treating illness. His own health challenge gave him the opportunity to experience what millions of cancer patients and their families experience. Because colostrum made such a difference in his healing journey, Dr. BeDell recommends daily supplementation to patients and friends who are facing serious health challenges. Colostrum helped his immune system return to a state of homeostasis so that his own body could heal him from within. Although not everyone is accepting of his advice, or not right away, Dr. BeDell shares his story with open-minded people who are ready to explore that which is beyond traditional medicine. He continues regular monitoring for pancreatic cancer with blood work and CT scans – all negative – and while he was once on twelve different medications, today, he doesn't take any and reports feeling healthier than he has in the last forty years. Additionally, after taking colostrum for those first six months and regularly working out at the gym, Dr. BeDell won first place in a power lifting contest for his age and weight category. Dr. BeDell welcomes people to connect with him through his website (bedell-chiro.com).

Tom White, Ph.C.
It's All About the Inflammation

Albuquerque pharmacist clinician and compounding pharmacist Tom White, Ph.C. is a unique type of medical practitioner by virtue of the fact that he practices in New Mexico. New Mexico is one of only three states with the highest level of credentialing that grants prescriptive authority from both the Medical Board and the Board of Pharmacy. This allows Dr. White the ability to assess, test, prescribe, and treat patients for hormone balance, anti-aging, and preventative medicine – in much the same way as a traditional medical doctor. TW Wellness Compounding Pharmacy offers patients a "one-stop" for their health needs. Dr. White has been in practice for more than three decades and is recognized as a pioneer in the field of Bio-Identical Hormone Therapy (BHRT).

Dr. White is committed to changing the health trajectory of his patients by reversing traditional medicine's treatment paradigm. He focuses on healing the gut and in turn, quelling the pervasive inflammation that is linked to nearly every major disease which brings patients to his office. At their initial visit, following a blood draw to measure key metabolic (insulin levels, fasting glucose, A1C) and inflammatory markers (C-reactive protein, Interleukin-6), patients participate in an in-depth consultation and education session. Dr. White believes that an educated patient will be a successful patient, so he spends time explaining how inflammation contributes to disease, why it's so dangerous, and how colostrum helps decrease inflammation. He tells them, "Inflammation is your biggest problem no matter what your problem is. When you start solving inflammation, you are going to live longer and you're going to be healthier."

Every patient leaves the pharmacy with a bag of powdered bovine colostrum and stern instructions to take it daily. And if those instructions go unheeded, Dr. White knows. Yes, Dr. White is the pharmacist who knows whether his patients have been good or not. After sixty days, he repeats the blood tests and if patients have been faithful to their colostrum regimen, the inflammatory markers go down and the metabolic markers improve. Patients typically feel better as their symptoms subside, but when they see substantial improvements from the pre- and post-test values, they know they're on the right track. Greater than 90% of patients choose to remain on colostrum as prescribed.

Dr. White's protocols have proved extremely efficacious. Nearly every one of his patients has experienced significant improvements in their overall daily functioning through the reduction in inflammation. He explains the reduction in systemic inflammation as a result of improved cortisol modulation, as it pertains to gut health. Contrary to what most people think about elevated cortisol levels being bad – often resulting from too much emotional stress – cortisol is a necessary hormone. As people age, the body's demand for cortisol increases, but the body's capacity for cortisol production decreases. A lot of inflammation begins in the gut, so by reducing gut inflammation, balancing the microbiome, and healing leaky gut, the body can then "bank" the cortisol for other metabolic reactions in the body. Dr. White believes that colostrum supplementation helps fix the G.I. issues that otherwise lead to an inefficient use of the patient's own dwindling cortisol production.

Keeping inflammation at bay is important at any age, but particularly important later in life, as is balancing the body's changing hormone production. Dr. White's area of expertise and bedside manner attract patients locally and from all fifty states who are seeking a solution to successful aging, reduced pain, and better health. To learn more Dr. White's practice of compounding pharmacy, BHRT, and how bovine colostrum calms inflammation, visit his website (tomwhitewellness.com).

Lucie Kotlářová, PharmDr.
Joining Forces Against Inflammation

As Director of InPharmClinic in the Czech Republic, clinical pharmacist Lucie Kotlářová, PharmDr. is focused on natural adjuvant treatments for remediating inflammation and strengthening the immune system in cancer patients. Dr. Kotlářová also treats patients with various conditions and generalized poor health stemming from immunocompromise, and she has noted a common thread in the thousands of patients she has helped over the years. Experience and research have taught her that poor nutrition, lifestyle, and environmental factors contribute to vitamin C deficiency which in turn, leads to impaired immunity. Immunocompromise increases infection susceptibility, probability of disease development, severity of organ failure, and mortality risk.

Vitamin C deficiency is exceedingly common in the United States and even more so in Dr. Kotlářová's native Czech Republic. Unlike other mammals, with the exception of guinea pigs, primates are unable to synthesize ascorbic acid in the liver due to a mutation in the gulonolactone oxidase (GULO) gene. So, unless dietary intake is abundantly sufficient – and this can be difficult to achieve – low plasma levels of ascorbic acid can lead to vitamin C deficiency and/or hypovitaminosis C (scurvy). The problem is compounded by the generation of reactive oxygen species (free radicals) by oxidative stress. It becomes part of the vicious cycle that leads to immunocompromise, and increases an individual's susceptibility to cancer and other immune-related conditions.

Vitamin C deficiency is also observed in critically ill patients with septic shock, often resulting from massive inflammation caused by a bowel infection (i.e., *C. difficile)* and leaky gut. Septic shock patients in the ICU experience hypovitaminosis C at a rate of nearly 40%, compared to the non-septic, still critically ill patients, at a rate of 25%.[111] Even when critically ill patients receive standard of care nutritional therapy, the rates of vitamin C deficiency can be as great as 75%.

Dr. Kotlářová believes addressing vitamin C deficiency with intravenous (I.V.) ascorbic acid is key to increasing a patient's chances of recovery and survival. Patients from the Czech Republic and surrounding countries come to her clinic for weekly infusions. Since the I.V. ascorbic acid can only be administered in the clinic, Dr. Kotlářová gives her patients an oral liposomal form of vitamin C to take daily between infusions. More recently, Dr. Kotlářová added bovine colostrum to her treatment protocols to better contend with inflammation, heal leaky gut, and promote immune resilience. Both vitamin C and colostrum impact immune function by enhancing the proliferation and differentiation of T-lymphocytes (T-cells) and B-lymphocytes (B-cells); stimulating natural killer (NK) cell activity; and modulating cytokine production. Vitamin C also provides powerful antioxidant activity against free radicals.

Vitamin C and bovine colostrum are two synergistic supplements that offer Dr. Kotlářová's patients a natural healing approach for their cancers, and many choose nutritional therapy as an adjunct to standard chemotherapy. In otherwise healthy people, Dr. Kotlářová views the combination of vitamin C and colostrum as a prevention strategy – one in which the immune system gets some extra help to fulfill its role of preventing viral infections and destroying random cancer cells which could potentially gain a foothold in the body. She recommends everyone supplement with oral vitamin C and bovine colostrum regardless of health status as the best way to defend against infections that might lead to serious immunocompromise. To learn more about Dr. Kotlářová or InPharmClinic, visit (inpharmclinic.cz).

Nicole Avena, Ph.D.
Blueprint for a Healthy Baby
There's a science to bringing healthy babies into the world and nurturing them towards adulthood and a lifetime of optimal health. Research neuroscientist and nutrition expert Nicole Avena, Ph.D. has helped create a nutritional blueprint for expectant mothers and fathers. As a public speaker and author, Dr. Avena has a unique opportunity to reach across the country – and literally, the world – to share her

message about diet during pregnancy as well as baby, toddler, and childhood nutrition. The sense of urgency may be more important now than ever as life expectancy among Americans, unrelated to the COVID-19 pandemic, has been gradually declining since 2014.[112]

Dr. Avena's blueprint entails pre-planning prior to baby's conception and throughout a couple's pregnancy with a focus on adequate and appropriate nutritional intake (i.e., vegetables, fruits, whole grains, and lean protein), and one that doesn't inadvertently cause nutritional deficiencies. Pregnant women and those intending to become pregnant can successfully follow vegetarian or vegan diets but should be cognizant of their overall nutritional intake. Restrictive diets or ones that exclude a specific food group are ill-advised because they can put undue stress on the mother-to-be, which in turn, affects her developing fetus. A general recommendation is a varied diet comprised of fresh or frozen whole foods and supplements recommended by one's OB/GYN, typically iron and folate. Dr. Avena believes that creating a solid foundation early is instrumental in tackling the exploding obesity epidemic and helping subsequent generations avoid the many ill health effects associated with being overweight or obese.

Breastfeeding is an integral part of the post-delivery plan, and Dr. Avena encourages mothers to breastfeed whenever possible. "Breast milk and colostrum are the perfect nutrition because they promote development of baby's body, brain, and immune system. Maternal antibodies strengthen a baby's immune system by establishing robust G.I. tract health which in turn, helps prevent future infections. Breastfeeding (and lack of) affects every aspect of development in babies, including mental development." Dr. Avena's strong advocacy for breastfeeding doesn't discount the fact that some women are unable to, or choose not to breastfeed. Ongoing advances have led to the creation of infant formulas that provide better nutrition and are more similar to breast-milk than in the past, but the all-important maternal anti-bodies in breastmilk and colostrum cannot be replicated.

Dr. Avena is also a strong breastfeeding advocate for its ability to foster the mother-baby bond during this critical time in a newborn's life. Close maternal relationships provide mental health benefits that carry into childhood and beyond. Extended breastfeeding – even beyond the six months recommended by the World Health Organization – adds to the bonding experience for both mother and baby. The skin-to-skin contact and baby's sucking boosts the mother's oxytocin levels which in turn, helps mom feel calm, drowsy and even euphoric; it also helps her uterus contract to its pre-pregnancy size. For baby, nursing and snuggling with mom stimulates oxytocin release which helps baby feel a sense of comfort and security.

In the situation that breastfeeding (or extended breast-feeding) is not an option, Dr. Avena recommends supple-mentation with processed bovine colostrum to enhance formula feeding. Bovine colostrum supplementation acts a surrogate in providing important immunoglobulins, anti-bodies, and a variety of immune-building components from a true mammalian source, which is closest to what's con-tained in mother's breastmilk. Dr. Avena is clear: "While nothing can replace breastmilk as the perfectly engineered food for babies, bovine colostrum may help fill some of the gaps left from formula feeding."

The effort and expense of having a child today is help-ing drive the quest for knowledge about all-things baby, and Dr. Avena credits the Internet with increasing the pub-lic's awareness about the benefits of breastfeeding and of colostrum specifically. Not only is basic information avail-able at one's fingertips 24/7, but when influencers take up the cause, the information is disseminated to a wider au-dience. The medical community's interest in infant health is also fueling clinical trials; at the present time, there are several investigations utilizing bovine colostrum as a fortifier to mother's milk in preterm infants.[113] If you or someone you love is pregnant or trying to become pregnant, visit Dr. Nicole Avena's website (drnicoleavena.com) for more information about having a healthy baby.

The human experience is filled with extraordinary events and circumstances that nudge us along in life, helping us to choose one path or another. Even when life seems utterly out of our control, personal choices are important, and the goal of making positive health choices contributes to a more fulfilling life. So, with the onslaught of autoimmune diseases, chronic health conditions, and more recently COVID-19, we need an action plan to improve G.I. health, which is key to a healthy immune system, a healthy brain, and robust health overall. So, here it is in three easy steps:

1) Claim your health sovereignty.
2) Adopt a heathier lifestyle.
3) Take powdered bovine colostrum daily.

It's really just that simple! Colostrum is truly the missing link to optimal physical health and mental well-being. No matter what eating style you adhere to – vegetarian, Mediterranean, DASH, Paleo, Keto, intermittent fasting, Kosher, or Halal – bovine colostrum can be an integral part of your nutrition. In fact, it should be the foundational part of your nutrition; any additional supplements may be added as needed. And if you're actively trying to lose weight and build muscle tissue, colostrum is absolutely necessary.

If you live in the spirit of the old saying, *an apple a day keeps the doctor away*, bovine colostrum redefines the medical profession. As nature's most basic and most effective "medicine," colostrum puts people on the path to immune resilience, reduced inflammation, and whole-body homeostasis which allows us to be our best selves in everything we choose to do in life. So, right now, I invite everyone to make a commitment to health sovereignty:

"I am responsible for my body. I am in control of my body. I shall take back my health. I shall strive to improve my health. I hereby assert my health sovereignty."

The Choice is Yours.
When You Have the Knowledge, You Have the Power to Heal Yourself.
Douglas A. Wyatt

9

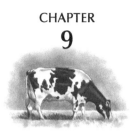

From Farm to Medicine Cabinet

Bringing bovine colostrum to the retail market was a labor of love. Only the people closest to me know otherwise. As with most memories of past experiences, hindsight makes them look and feel a whole lot better, and twenty-five years ago – well, that's a lot of hindsight. The reality was that it was at times, emotionally strained as Kaye and I attempted to navigate the retail environment. We felt blessed to have been given the opportunity to share our rediscovery of colostrum with people who needed its healing qualities. My marketing background was definitely an asset, and Kaye's storytelling was compelling, yet neither of us had any real experience in launching a retail product. We did, of course, have some very talented and hardworking people who truly believed in colostrum's ability to improve health, helping us along the way. As Symbiotics grew to accommodate more employees, we expanded our messaging outreach. We did quite well early on when colostrum was a hot, new supplement and popular with athletes and body builders, thanks in part to the clinical studies involving Australian athletes. Our colostrum sold well in the smaller health food stores and independent grocery stores, but we always contended with the expense of acquiring prime shelf space. These costs increased with each passing year and became nearly unsustainable.

In the early days, Symbiotics sold colostrum in capsule form (later, it became available in powdered form). The rationale was two-fold. First, people love to take pills for convenience sake. I tend to think of it as a pill obsession, and Americans seem to have a higher degree of it than other cultures – take a multi-vitamin once a day instead of getting the RDAs from five to eight servings of fruits and vegetables. This is a bit of a generalization, but it parallels the "magic bullet" approach to getting healthier, for example: "Can't I just take a pill and lose weight?" Second, capsular form allowed the colostrum to reach further down the G.I. tract before the gelatin capsule dissolved. The capsule afforded some protection from the overly harsh acidic environment of the stomach. If more of colostrum's immune bioactives and growth factors could make it intact to the small intestine, the better, and more would be absorbed into the bloodstream.

When colostrum comes directly from the mammary gland, every droplet is surrounded by a protective lipid membrane, so if you drank raw, fresh liquid colostrum from a cow, goat, or sheep, it would transit intact to the small intestine. However, during the manufacturing of colostrum supplements, this membrane is fractured, which in turn, results in digestion of the colostrum in the stomach (i.e., breakdown into amino acids). With the loss of the protective membrane, the colostrum is less effective as it relates to the actual measured quantity. In other words, you would need more of the powdered colostrum to achieve the desired effect(s). This was observed in the early athletic research, which determined sixty grams as the necessary dosage to elicit an effect on performance.

This situation presented a unique problem which persisted for a number of years, and so Symbiotics sold capsules exclusively until a solution could be realized. The nagging question: *What if there was a way to restore the lipid membrane that was fractured during the manufacturing process?* In the early 2000s, I commissioned two of the leading scientists at the Paris-Sorbonne University to develop a lipid-based formula and application process which would effectively restore a functioning lipid membrane to the colostrum, and mimic the lipid membrane on fresh, raw, liquid colostrum. This new "lipid delivery" technology protected the bioactives from stomach acids, thereby increasing the amount of bioactives available for entry into the cells.

Most clinical trials at the time utilized 60 grams of colostrum per day, but I felt that with liposomal delivery, it stood to reason that a lower dose could be just as effective. I commissioned a double-blind clinical trial which showed liposomal colostrum could elicit desired results with just 20 grams per day instead of 60 grams.[114] Most studies today utilize a dose of 20 grams, which also turns out to be a cost-savings benefit for athletes. Bovine colostrum has the distinction of being the first nutritional supplement to utilize this technology, and our proprietary LD Liposomal Delivery™ has been a gamechanger in the colostrum industry.

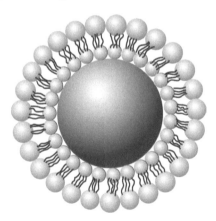

Figure 4 – The Bilayer Structure of a Liposome

Aside from increased effectiveness, another significant advantage of our LD Liposomal Delivery™ is that when powdered colostrum mixed with water is ingested, the action begins immediately in the mouth. The immune bioactives can go to work on the oral microbiome and once swallowed, more of the G.I. real estate benefits. This increases the number of conditions that can be impacted by colostrum's healing capabilities – gingivitis, heartburn, GERD, and general esophageal irritation. Furthermore, absorption of the proline-rich polypeptides (PRPs) occurs primarily in the back of the throat and sublingually, something that is bypassed with capsules. Consumers still utilize capsules for convenience, yet I advocate more for powder and once people understand the rationale, they agree.

Lipid delivery technology remained elusive for other supplement companies and as I detailed in Chapter 5, some brought cheaper, lower IgG-content, (and less effective) colostrum brands to the market. This irresponsible, profit-driven strategy tanked the whole colostrum supplement industry. Consumers went to health food stores and reached for the cheapest brand, believing that it was all the same quality, and when they failed to get results, they stopped buying. As brick-and-mortar businesses began migrating to online sales, I dipped my toes in the water, but the water was way too cold, and I pulled back. In 2004, I sold Symbiotics to Naturade (as of 2020, it's Prevention, LLC dba Naturade).

Then tragedy struck in 2006 when Kaye died from throat cancer. She waged a valiant fight until the very end, as did many people who underwent thymus radiation in childhood and suffered a similar fate. We were thankful for the time we had together, and I truly believe that if it had not been for our rediscovery of colostrum, my personal loss would have been years earlier. Despite my tsunami of grief, Kaye is never far from my mind, and one of the ways I honor her is by telling her story at every opportunity. Even in death, Kaye gives hope to those who need it most – those who need a healing miracle. Yet, I needed something, too – perhaps a distraction from my grief, but that was difficult to come by.

In the two years after I sold Symbiotics, I did some serious self-reflection when it came to how I wanted to move forward. When I was finally ready to throw myself back into the business world, I could have gone in any direction but found myself once again being guided towards colostrum. The concept of health sovereignty inspired me to register both the company name (Sovereign Laboratories) and domain name (SovereignLaboratories.com) for future use. Certainly, I knew the colostrum industry well, but this time, the motivation was different; it came from healthcare professionals, their patients, and everyday consumers who'd found my telephone number in the phone book or my email address somewhere. They'd tell me how the colostrum they currently took just didn't work as well, and asked if I would consider getting back into the business. Once I realized these calls and emails weren't simply one-offs, I knew that it was right time for a new chapter.

This time around, the prospect of selling in brick-and-mortar stores was a definite "no," and I found myself ready for another dip into the pool of online sales. Convinced that this would be the future of retail sales, I wanted to be a part of it, so I needed to *just do it*. I started in the shallow end (i.e., my home office) with a simple website, selling a few products under the "New Life Colostrum" brand name. This new world of online sales was perfect for me because I was able to keep minimal expenses, keep my own hours, and keep in touch with colostrum users. As the business began to grow, I waded out a little further and by 2012, Sovereign Laboratories launched its signature powdered bovine colostrum supplement – Colostrum-LD®. (In retrospect, registering the domain a few years earlier was a god-send.) With the help of a few former Symbiotics employees and some bright new talent, the next decade was primed for success.

Sovereign Laboratories experienced tremendous growth in the following years, and our product line expanded to include other bovine colostrum-based products for G.I. and immune health. I set my sights on attending professional conferences which ran the gamut from traditional medicine to functional medicine to chiropractic to anti-aging and nutrition. The goal was to introduce as many people in the healthcare arena to colostrum so that they could, at least, explore it as a therapy for patients for whom "regular" modalities did not help. My messaging was, however, much wider: Every patient who walks through your door with any sort of complaint needs bovine colostrum. With the ever-expanding use of social media, I reached out to health-minded influencers and colostrum advocates to share their experiences and bring my message directly to consumers. Being in the middle of the pool was both personally and professionally rewarding.

By 2019, I relinquished the day-to-day running of Sovereign Laboratories and turned my focus to the Vibrant Life Institute (VLI), a 501(3)(c) non-profit organization dedicated to colostrum education, safe food advocacy, and health sovereignty. In the same way that other free thinkers go across the grain, VLI enables me to get my message across without unnecessary bureaucratic entanglement. I feel the message of colostrum is too powerful and too important to be compromised in any way. Yet, colostrum is not the singular solution I hoped it could be – or may have been in simpler times. And for all the good daily colostrum supplementation can do, it is only a stop-gap measure. The pervasive use of glyphosate, antibiotics, and other toxins is stymieing our collective health, and we must take a stand against it if we are to protect future generations. These man-made antagonists that were once sold to us as "modern progress" will continue to erode our bodies, making us more susceptible to infections.

Prior to publication – mid-2021, COVID-19 had taken more than 600,000 American lives and was responsible for 3.9 million deaths worldwide.[115] With two of every 100 COVID-positive Americans dying of COVID-related complications, the need for immune resilience is more important than ever before. I fervently believe that bovine colostrum plays an instrumental role in sufficiently modulating the immune system so it is at the ready to fight SARS-CoV-2 and prevents the debilitating and deadly cytokine storm observed in COVID-19. The hypothesis is that colostrum's antiviral activity is similar to the efficacy demonstrated against influenza and other viruses.[116,117] The likely mechanisms of action are via immunoglobulins and natural killer (NK) cell activation.[118,119] Because all viruses including SARS-CoV-2 are subject to mutation, NK cells provide a viable defense, unlike commercial vaccines that may become outdated and less effective as the virus mutates.

Furthermore, now that SARS-CoV-2 has been circulating the globe for at least 18 months, it is not unreasonable to believe that dairy cows are generating antibodies to some or all of the variants. Remember: Cows can produce antibodies to human diseases while not becoming infected themselves, just by virtue of being around people who are infected. As I've described previously in relation to the origins of vaccine development, bovine antibody production to predominantly human diseases is not a new phenomenon. Humankind has relied on this type of symbiotic relationship with the bovine since they were first domesticated. Cows are quite literally "walking, natural pharmacies," from which both we and our pets can reap the benefits.

The concept of bovine antibodies against SARS-CoV-2 has already begun to appear in the scientific literature and has been offered as a potential therapeutic opportunity.[120,121,122] It may also be possible to elicit antibody production by inoculating female cows with SARS-CoV-2; this is commonly known as hyperimmune colostrum. Intentional inoculation simply speeds up the process and can be targeted to a specific variant.

In the current COVID-19 crisis, we have several factors working against us – extreme contagiousness, inability to halt the spread, a lack of healthcare resources, no widely available monoclonal antibody treatment, lingering debilitation and vaccine hesitancy. So, if and until herd immunity can be achieved, I remind you of Hippocrates words, "Let food be thy medicine." A return to our not-so-distant past, when bovine colostrum and milk supplied our antibiotics and antivirals, may just be what's needed to create immune resilience and homeostasis in the body. It qualifies as a "do no harm" approach, does not require a prescription, and is now garnering attention as a potential therapeutic for emerging viral threats.[123,124]

Clinical trials sponsored by New Image™ International are set to begin soon with my old friend Graeme Clegg at the helm. His team will be investigating colostrum as a tool for the management of respiratory coronaviruses. We eagerly await the results, as this potentially represents the first nutrition-based immune supplement that could become available on a mass scale at very low cost. But until then, who exactly needs bovine colostrum? Even pre-COVID, when I was asked this question, my answer was "Absolutely everyone!" That advice just might be more important now.

A Guide to Determining Whether You Should Take Colostrum

1. Do you regularly use aspirin, NSAIDs, or prescription pain medications?
2. Do you regularly use over-the-counter or prescription anti-acids?
3. Have you had a course of oral antibiotics in the previous three years?
4. Do you have any food allergies or intolerances, including lactose intolerance?
5. Do you have allergies or asthma?
6. Do you suffer with a chronic or autoimmune disease?
7. Do you have arthritis or joint pain?
8. Do you have G.I. conditions such as Crohn's disease, irritable bowel syndrome (IBS), ulcerative colitis, or stomach/small intestine ulcers?
9. Have you been diagnosed with leaky gut?
10. Has bloodwork indicated elevated markers or inflammation (C-reactive protein, Interleukin-6)?
11. Do you have impaired glucose tolerance, or have you been diagnosed with diabetes or prediabetes?
12. Are you twenty or more pounds above your ideal body weight?
13. Are you an alcoholic?
14. Do you live in a highly toxic environment (air pollution, contaminated water)?
15. Were you breastfed for less than one year?

A YES answer to any one or more of the above questions means you should definitely be taking colostrum.

In addition to general G.I. and immune health, these are the most common uses I advocate for bovine colostrum:

➤ In patients with any type of allergy or autoimmune condition, colostrum can heal and prevent leaky gut syndrome, and halt and reverse the destruction of the corresponding tissue or organs caused by inflammation and autoimmunity.

➤ For athletes, colostrum can help shorten recovery time following intense exercise; build lean muscle mass; burn adipose tissue; maintain ideal blood glucose levels; accelerate healing of injuries; preserve and boost immune function; and heal leaky gut.

➤ To combat the deleterious effects associated with human aging, colostrum can help enhance health and healing from chronic diseases, including arthritis, osteoporosis, type 2 diabetes, heart disease, cancer, depression, and various types of neurocognitive decline.

➤ For patients with chronic pain, colostrum helps reduce the inflammation that precipitates painful joints, muscles and connective tissue, thereby reducing reliance on dangerous pain medications.

➤ For arthritis sufferers, colostrum helps tone down the body's inflammatory response by healing leaky gut syndrome, which halts the erosion of joint tissue; and helps rebuild joint tissue.

➤ To address skin conditions and minor topical wounds, colostrum's growth factors help promote repair and regeneration of skin cells; healing leaky gut helps resolve inflammatory-related skin eruptions such as acne, rosacea, psoriasis.

➤ To fight superbugs and avoid antibiotic use, colostrum contains antibodies to the disease-causing pathogens the cow has encountered in her lifetime as well as those received from her mother.

➤ To fight influenza and other viral infections, colostrum's PRPs stimulate the human immune system to fight microbial pathogens and to develop antibodies soon after exposure.

➤ In dieters and patients with diabetes, pre-diabetes or metabolic syndrome, colostrum can assist in weight loss by increasing lean body mass; increasing metabolism; increasing insulin sensitivity; regulating blood glucose and leptin levels; decreasing appetite; and detoxifying the body.

➤ For infants who are not breastfed, colostrum's growth factors help promote gut maturation and avoid leaky gut; along with immunoglobulins and other immune bioactives, growth factors encourage healthy growth and development, especially in preterm and non-thriving infants.

➤ In the post-partum woman, colostrum can help the new mom return to her pre-pregnancy fitness level; avoid respiratory infections; re-establish robust bowel and vaginal heath; and improve overall health and mental well-being.

➤ For individuals struggling with mild mental health issues, colostrum can help instill calmness, improve mood, and support psychological well-being.

➤ In mammalian pets, colostrum supports a healthy immune system; aids in digestion and balances gut bacteria; sustains energy levels; increases lean body mass; and stimulates healthy skin and coat.

In the next chapter, I'll discuss the uses of colostrum in more detail. Healthcare practitioners from various specialties will share how their patients benefit from bovine colostrum supplementation. And if you haven't already, as I invited you in Chapter 8, ...to choose to live a life of maximum healthspan.*

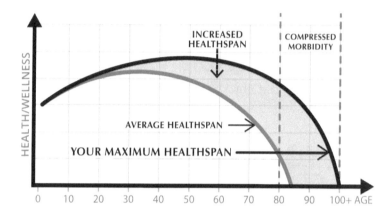

Figure 5: Increased Healthspan and Compressed Morbidity

*Healthspan refers to the concept of living longer (more years) without a major chronic disease(s). Any illness comes at the end of life and thus, the period of suffering is minimal.

10

The Ultimate Superfood for People and Their Pets

It's been called a superfood, a medical food, liquid gold, and Mother Nature's healing miracle, and people have been using it as a dietary supplement to improve athletic performance, promote healthy aging, knock down inflammation, restore gut health, and optimize immune function for centuries. However you refer to colostrum, or if you're learning about it just now, please don't call it "too good to be true." From the anthropology perspective, colostrum is the one nutritional substance to guarantee a mammalian species' survival. As a human dietary supplement, there is no other "superfood" more versatile than colostrum. Period.

The one thing colostrum has not been called is a drug – and for good reason. Unlike drugs, colostrum does not have a long list of side effects and warnings associated with it. Bovine colostrum has achieved GRAS (Generally Recognized as Safe) status; this designation means that it can be incorporated into consumer foods and beverages. Of course, its health benefits are more readily realized when liposomal colostrum is consumed with only pure water. The only potential downside to regular colostrum consumption – if you can call it that – is the increase in villi height in the small intestine. The villi (finger-like projections) are responsible for increasing the surface area in the small intestine so that micronutrients from digested food can be absorbed into the bloodstream.

We have observed in piglets that when you feed them hydrochloric acid, the villi are greatly damaged; their height is reduced which negatively affects nutrient absorption. However, if you feed the piglets colostrum, the villi grow back and even gain an extra twenty percent in height.[125] In humans, an increase in villi height increases the absorption of nutrients as well as any oral medications you might be taking, which may lead to a more pronounced effect of that drug(s). Certain drugs may seem "more effective" when patients are also taking colostrum on a regular basis. In this case, I recommend patients speak to their physicians to determine whether a change in the medication dosage is necessary to obtain the desired or anticipated effect.

The rationale behind one's decision to take colostrum can be influenced by a variety of factors – whether it's a recommendation from a healthcare provider or something they've read online or print, or from the childbirth/childrearing experience itself. People generally have one or more specific reasons depending on their current health status and desired results. Even healthcare practitioners recommend colostrum based on their own experience or field of expertise. My argument is that you can't go wrong taking colostrum and that we all need its immune bioactives and growth factors to achieve and maintain optimal health and well-being.

What follows are practitioners' accounts of the various uses for which they recommend bovine colostrum supplementation and are true testament to colostrum's healing capabilities.

GASTROINTESTINAL HEALTH
Donald R. Henderson, M.D. – *Early Adopter of an Ancient Medicine*

Like many medical professionals, Los Angeles gastroen-terologist Donald R. Henderson, M.D. was initially skeptical about bovine colostrum. As a "traditional" doctor, his practice was defined by procedures – colonoscopies and cauterizations for hemorrhoids, bowel obstructions, ulcers, intestinal bleeding, and cancers. And like many of Dr. Henderson's colleagues, there was hardly any nutrition education included in medical training in the 1970s, and certainly no "alternative" healthcare. A chance encounter with Kaye changed him into a believer, and so not only was Dr. Henderson an early adopter of colostrum supplementation but a true champion. He and Kaye later went on to co-author a book, *Colostrum: Nature's Healing Miracle.* Dr. Henderson recommended colostrum to patients with all types of conditions, not just those related to his specialty. Through study and experience, he found colostrum to be a safe and effective supplement for patients of all ages with colitis, Crohn's disease, gastritis, and other G.I. disorders – many of whom also suffered with rheumatoid arthritis, asthma, and allergies.

Dr. Henderson was intrigued by bovine colostrum for its potential use against the growing number of antibiotic-resistant infections that had become all too prevalent. He was alarmed by the shrinking number of antibiotics that remained effective against the most serious bacterial infections, which had resulted from indiscriminate and inappropriate use by his profession. Also on the forefront of his mind were the environmental assaults that stressed the immune system. Many of Dr. Henderson's patients heralded from Los Angeles County and were regularly exposed to cigarette smoke, vehicle exhaust fumes, air pollution, contaminated drinking water, radiation, and pesticide residues in low-quality foods. He realized that these poisons were making his very young and elderly patients more susceptible to opportunistic infections, chronic diseases and disability, and in turn, reducing their quality of life.

Dr. Henderson often described the bioactives in colostrum as "little policeman" who surveilled the intestinal tract for cancerous cells. In the absence of a perfectly functioning immune system, these bioactives could destroy the cancer cells before they had a chance to rapidly grow and metastasize beyond the G.I. tract. Colostrum was the one all-natural supplement he could offer patients to support the immune system and protect against a high-mortality cancer. Sadly, Donald R. Henderson, M.D. passed away in 2020. He was a true credit to his profession and in my mind, a lifesaver for educating his patients about colostrum.

INTEGRATIVE HEALTHCARE
Weston "Wiggy" Saunders, M.D. – *A Holistic Approach to Medicine*

Family medicine doctor, Weston "Wiggy" Saunders, M.D. embraced his calling to integrative medicine early on during medical school, and his patients in Winston-Salem, North Carolina and the surrounding area now reap the benefits. Identifying and addressing underlying health conditions within the context of a whole-person approach not only gets results, but it shows patients that they are more than just a named disease with a prescription(s) to fill. Dr. Saunders draws from his personal experience with adrenal fatigue to develop rapport with patients, which he believes is critical to patient success. Dr. Saunders also goes further to distinguish between *normal* health and *optimal* health, and he works with patients to optimize their health potential so they can live their best life. His practice, Robinhood

Integrative Health, embodies a holistic, people-oriented approach to medical care, and every team member follows the "health as it ought to be" motto envisioned by Dr. Saunders.

Dr. Saunders treats a wide range of autoimmune diseases, allergies, hormonal imbalances, and chronic microbial infections (i.e., Epstein-Barr virus, Lyme disease, Mycoplasma, mold toxicity). New patients from across the age spectrum come to his practice, often with multiple conditions and having suffered for years without relief, or even a proper diagnosis from traditional medicine. Dr. Saunders attributes stress, leaky gut, toxicity, hormone/thyroid imbalances, and immune system dysfunction for many of the conditions plaguing people today.

For most people, the first step in the healing process is fixing the gut. Dr. Saunders often puts his patients on a gut restoration protocol that includes bovine colostrum. With this protocol, patients' immune health and symptoms greatly improve. Successful patient outcomes have made Dr. Saunders a strong proponent of bovine colostrum who refers to it as a "wonderfood." In this regard, Dr. Saunders is part of a new generation of medical doctors seeking natural ways to use nutrition and lifestyle as healing modalities to combat the ill effects of modern life. To learn more about bovine colostrum's role in integrative medicine and Dr. Wiggy Saunders' family medicine practice, visit RobinhoodIntegrativeHealth.com.

Heidi Iratcabal, N.D. – *Colostrum as Code*
As a naturopath for more than two decades, Heidi Iratcabal, N.D. began utilizing bovine colostrum after hearing a lecture given by world renown colostrum expert Andrew Keech, Ph.D. Dr. Iratcabal now incorporates bovine colos-

trum in her treatment protocols to help patients who suffer with gastrointestinal issues, joint or chronic pain, and a multitude of conditions involving immune dysregulation or immunocompromise. Her integrative medical practice, Carpathia Collaborative, located in Dallas, Texas, offers patient-centered solutions designed to promote life-long health optimization. The name 'Carpathia' refers to the only passenger ship that attempted to rescue passengers from the Titanic, and so it's a metaphor for Dr. Iratcabal's goal to help save patients from the sinking model of conventional medicine.

While most of Dr. Iratcabal's patients know what colostrum is per say, they're all surprised when she tells them that colostrum can support immune health in adulthood. And Dr. Iratcabal has found a unique way of educating her patients about the immune benefits and why taking colostrum becomes more important as people age and develop immune challenges. "Colostrum is the 'coded material' that signals the immune system, specifically, the cytokines, to turn on and begin learning about life outside the womb. The normal cytokine signals become dysregulated with advancing age and/or with a state of immunocompromise, so taking colostrum daily helps reboot and rebalance those signals." Patients typically notice changes in their health within a few weeks as their bodies begin to recover their normal (and healthy) functioning. Dr. Iratcabal's Crohn's patients have experienced great relief by taking bovine colostrum; when the frequency and severity of flare-ups decrease, patients have been able to reduce the amount of medications they take.

Dr. Iratcabal also works with professional and amateur athletes who find colostrum beneficial for increasing muscle strength and improving recovery between workouts. As an athlete who monitors her own health carefully, Dr. Iratcabal attests to colostrum's effect on exercise recovery and more consistent energy levels from day to day. It's her go-to functional food at the first sign of illness and helps reset her body after long periods of travel and/or changes in her normal sleep schedule. If you would like to learn more about Heidi Iratcabal, N.D.'s integrative approach to healthcare, visit CarpathiaCollaborative.com.

Alicia Galvin, R.D. – *Food as Thy Medicine*

Registered dietitian Alicia Galvin has the unique opportunity to connect with patients in the Texas communities of Dallas and Fort Worth. Not only does she see referrals from a multitude of medical specialties – G.I., internal medicine, allergy and immunology, and dermatology – she is able to spend more quality time educating them about the importance of good nutrition. Bovine colostrum supplementation may not be part of the standard educational program for dietitians, but it certainly appeals to early adopters such as Ms. Galvin who learned about colostrum from a colleague. The wide-reaching benefits of colostrum supplementation make it ideal for most, if not all, the health conditions that dietitians address with their clients, including Crohn's disease, ulcerative colitis, celiac disease, Hashimoto's thyroiditis, psoriasis, and eczema.

Ms. Galvin is also a proponent of bovine colostrum for treating symptoms that arise from Lyme disease and mold toxicity, which are being diagnosed more frequently today. She sees the effects of increased intestinal permeability (i.e., allergies, extreme food sensitivities, acute episodes of diarrhea, GERD) on a patient's quality of life and recommends colostrum as the starting point to improve gut health. Those with GERD and/or acute diarrhea show the most impressive results with symptoms easing or disappearing within two to three days. Because bowel functioning is such a critical aspect of human physiology, patients often seek the help of a registered dietitian when bowel issues arise, even something as "minor" as diarrhea triggered by food poisoning (i.e., a gut infection). In cases such as this, Ms. Galvin recommends increasing the frequency of colostrum until the diarrhea subsides and then adding foods back in slowly. Patients with autoimmune conditions, Lyme disease, or allergies take longer to feel relief – from several weeks to a few months. Ms. Galvin stresses to clients that colostrum is not a magic bullet, but taking it consistently over time with appropriate dietary modifications, offers a natural, non-pharmacological approach to chronic disease management – something that many clients prefer. Colostrum embodies her treatment philosophy: "A therapeutic approach to food is to view it as medicine for the body — restore balance, heal and produce vitality." If you would like to connect with Alicia Galvin, R.D., visit AliciaGalvinRD.com.

CHIROPRACTIC CARE
Mark Pederson, D.C. – *More Than Just an Adjustment*
Mark Pederson, D.C. shatters the notion that chiropractic is simply about spinal manipulation. His Warren, Minnesota practice, Optimal Health Family Chiropractic, offers comprehensive health and wellness services with a focus on therapies for leaky gut and autoimmune conditions, as he blends aspects of Western and Eastern medicine. Dr. Pederson's passion for a whole-person approach to care stems from his post-doctoral training in nutrition, neurology, and functional medicine, and his patients' good health reflects his twenty-five years of expertise and experience. His guiding philosophy is that the human body is continually working to repair and heal itself, and the chiropractor's job is to assist in whichever modalities work best for the

individual patient.

Initially, a majority of Dr. Pederson's patients come in due to an inflammatory-related condition such as an auto accident, a slip and fall, or a sports injury, and in the treatment of these conditions, Dr. Pederson often identifies systemic inflammation related to lifestyle and chronic diseases. He recommends daily supplementation with bovine colostrum to knock down both systemic and localized inflammation, to which he attests quicker and better patient outcomes. For localized areas of pain, such as a sprained ankle, Dr. Pederson uses powdered colostrum as a topical therapy pack so the anti-inflammatory bioactives can penetrate the skin directly. Patients experiencing this for the first time are quite surprised with their results, as was Dr. Pederson when he first noticed that colostrum could perform this way.

Prior to Dr. Pederson's introduction to bovine colostrum, he utilized the 4R/5R nutritional approach to treating leaky gut and autoimmune conditions – Remove the gut stressors. Replace digestive secretions. Re-inoculate with good bacteria. Repair gut lining with vitamin, minerals, omega-3 fish oils. Rebalance lifestyle choices. He found that patients' symptoms waxed and waned, but never fully resolved. By adding colostrum, patients improved greatly, and it's become the foundational supplement for all of Dr. Pederson's intestinal healing/anti-inflammatory protocols. He likens bovine colostrum to a superfood rather than a simple supplement because he's witnessed the benefits of health and vitality in so many of his patients. For additional information about Mark Pederson, D.C. and his family chiropractic practice, visit Optimal-Health.co.

ATHLETIC PERFORMANCE & FITNESS
Michele Neil Sherwood, D.O. and Mark Sherwood, N.D.
– Functional Medicine Fitness Gurus

Tulsa, Oklahoma physicians Michele Neil Sherwood, D.O. and Mark Sherwood, N.D. are trailblazers in wellness medicine and focus their patients' care around individualized treatment protocols. They've adopted a whole-person approach to medical care, and patients benefit from a comprehensive approach which spans the gamut of the duo's medical expertise – anti-aging, naturopathic, and functional medicine, osteopathic manipulative therapy, and lifestyle coaching. Patients learn the importance of nutrition, medical food and supplementation, exercise and functional movement, rest, stress management, and hormone balance. Both doctors have a background in athletics and physical fitness which makes them living role models to patients and clients of all ages, particularly the over 50s.

The Drs. Sherwood are committed to helping people achieve true healing by (1) eradicating self-imposed, choice-driven disease conditions, and (2) eliminating the usage of unnecessary medications. In other words, health sovereignty. Their vision to change the worldwide healthcare crisis one person at a time reaches beyond their Functional Medical Institute in Tulsa; television audiences across the Midwest U.S. can tune in to their weekly show. As physique title holders, the Drs. Sherwood are big proponents of bovine colostrum – twenty to twenty-five grams daily – for its ability to build lean muscle tissue and improve the overall appearance of their bodies.

Over the last ten years, the Drs. Sherwood have seen a lot of patients who want to become healthier and to look good as they start getting older and begin noticing changes in their physical appearance. Many also have some degree of immunocompromise or an autoimmune condition, so colostrum supplementation complements both goals. Initially, the doctors find themselves educating patients as to what colostrum is – "nature's first food." When patients see and feel results (i.e., less gas, bloating, abdominal pain and improved digestion) within the first few weeks, they're more likely to stick with the lifestyle changes that the doctors prescribe. By optimizing the immune system and improving overall gastrointestinal function, patients are better able to direct their newly increased energy levels to their workouts. To learn more about the importance of bovine colostrum in functional medicine, visit the Functional Medical Institute at FMIDR.com.

WOUND HEALING
Tom White, Ph.C. – *A Wound Healing Success Story*
Like many practitioners, there was for pharmacist clinician and compounding pharmacist Tom White, Ph.C., a time "BC" – *Before Colostrum*. For more than four decades, Dr. White has served the people of Albuquerque and the surrounding areas by helping them become healthy and feel better. When he was introduced to bovine colostrum at an anti-aging medical conference, he gained an appreciation for colostrum as a new modality to manage inflammation and treat gut dysbiosis. He now prescribes powdered bovine colostrum for everyone he treats, and results have been overwhelmingly positive and, in some cases, extraordinarily dramatic.

One of Dr. White's patients called him with an urgent problem; her ninety-year-old father had stumbled and landed quite hard. The damage to his forearm was severe, and the ICU attending physician was convinced that the combination of Coumadin® therapy that the patient was on and the injury sustained in the fall would most likely lead to his premature demise. Dr. White was familiar with wound research involving topical use of colostrum, so he recommended that the wound care specialist irrigate the wound with saline followed by a light dusting of powdered colostrum before bandaging the arm. This process was performed daily, and the patient also began taking two times the recommended daily dose of colostrum orally. Within three weeks, the patient's arm had completely healed.

Despite some initial resistance, the wound care specialist gained valuable insight and a new modality to use with future patients. The transforming growth factors (TGF-α and TGF-β) and epithelial growth factor (EGF) in colostrum help stimulate topical wound healing, and the oral colostrum provides an added healing boost. Clinical trials with colostrum powder dressings show that in addition to faster healing of deep wounds, patients experience less pain, more compliance, and a fewer number of dressings are required compared to conventional dressings.[126] That experience helped solidify Dr. White's approach to topical wounds in his own patients. To learn more about Dr. White's practice, TW Wellness Compounding Pharmacy & Clinic, visit his website (TomWhiteWellness.com).

VETERINARY USE & PET HEALTH
Todd Metcalf, D.V.M. – *Holistic Healthcare for Fur Babies*
Holistic veterinarian Todd Metcalf, D.V.M. is a treasured asset in the small rural community of Sedona, Arizona that he serves. Like many of the pet parents who themselves seek out complementary and alternative care for their own health, their furry pets receive care that adheres to a mind/body approach. Dr. Metcalf has been practicing

veterinary medicine for nearly four decades of which the last seventeen have incorporated holistic care. He offers personalized integrative care to Sedona's dogs and cats and helps them transition from a state of mental discord and physical disease to a state of mental well-being and physical health.

Dr. Metcalf utilizes a combination of natural techniques, including acupuncture, chiropractic, herbs, and nutritional therapy, to complement traditional veterinary medicine. He also incorporates powdered bovine colostrum into the treatment plan for conditions that require G.I. healing, microbiome restoration, immunity enhancement, and topical wound healing. Dr. Metcalf finds that colostrum is especially beneficial for underweight, non-thriving kittens who did not receive their mother's colostrum, and he recommends mixing the bovine colostrum with goat's milk rather than formula for better digestibility. Since dogs frequently suffer from the same digestive-related problems as humans (i.e., leaky gut, gut dysbiosis), bovine colostrum is a natural remedy that is very appealing to owners who see their pets' health improve quite dramatically in a relatively short period of time.

Dr. Metcalf has been a proponent of bovine colostrum supplementation for well over a dozen years and takes colostrum because he feels that it does his body good. He also keeps up with the professional veterinary literature on colostrum as well as human studies and understands the universality of bovine colostrum for other mammals. Many of Dr. Metcalf's patients are the sole companions for their elderly owners, so he's committed to helping their fur babies live longer, healthier lives filled with endless energy and vitality. So, in a sense, Dr. Metcalf cares for two sets of patients – the ones with fur and the ones without. To learn more about holistic veterinary care, visit the website for Dr. Metcalf's practice, Sunshine Holistic Veterinary Services (SunshineHolisticVet.com).

Now, a big question for many is: *How much colostrum do I need to take to get results like these?* The answer is: It depends. The amount of colostrum the human body needs is influenced by several factors, including present health condition, age, weight and body composition, lifestyle factors, and of course, the desired results. I recommend preventive, therapeutic, and maintenance doses and encourage individuals to find the level of use that provides them optimal results. Since most people taking colostrum are also in-tune with their bodies, the dosing is easy to determine based on how they feel – body and mind. Because colostrum is a food and not a drug, the term "dosing" really isn't accurate, but since it's the terminology that most people understand, I will address colostrum dosing in the next chapter.

11

The Health Sovereignty Solution

Just about everyone and their uncles (aunts, too) has written a book, published a blog, or given podcast testimony to the benefits of a particular diet, exercise regime, detox protocol, mind enhancing strategy, natural disease cure, or some "secret" to make all your health woes go away. And while the specific details change over time, the one consistency is the underlying concept that individuals have the power to make a change(s) in their own lives if they choose to do so. I didn't write this book to tell you to give up Fruit A in favor of Fruit B or to eat Vegetable A while running backwards every other day of the week. My purpose is to share my knowledge about colostrum through research, practitioners' experience, industry experts, and my personal story with Kaye. Health sovereignty relies upon knowledge. Armed with knowledge, YOU can make decisions that positively impact your health and the health of your dependent family members (and pets, too). You can also share that knowledge with others.

So, we come to the question on everyone's minds: *How much colostrum should I be taking?* First, I want to be exceeding clear that taking colostrum every day is not a substitute for an unhealthy lifestyle. Aside from being over-fed (i.e., overweight, obese), a majority of Americans are undernourished, and because their daily nutrition lacks the high-quality micronutrients, they aren't able to function at their highest potential, but colostrum is not a silver bullet. You can't smoke or drink excessively or eat fast food every day and believe that colostrum will cancel out the cellular and tissue damage to your heart, lungs, liver, brain, and the like. You must make a commitment to the habits that we know to be heath-enhancing – nutritious eating, regular exercise, quality sleep, mental stimulation, tobacco abstinence, and alcohol moderation. Yet, if you are a former smoker, a recovering alcoholic, or a reformed fast-food junkie, colostrum offers hope for renewal of your body systems. Colostrum's growth factors (*See Chapter 4.*) assist in this regard.

As I mentioned previously, the amount of colostrum necessary is a subjective measure and determined by several individual factors (i.e., present health condition, age, weight and body composition, lifestyle factors). It has been my experience over the past two decades – based on what patients and doctors tell me – is that most people achieve results with relatively small amounts of powdered colostrum when they use it consistently. If you live a "clean" life, these are my recommendations for everyone over the age of two:

Preventive Dosing / General Need: 1 teaspoon twice a day
This dose would be for an otherwise healthy person who does not have obvious symptoms or a diagnosis of a chronic or autoimmune disease and/or wants to protect against leaky gut and maintain a healthy gut microbiome and G.I. tract.

Therapeutic / Advanced Need: 2 teaspoons twice a day
This dose is intended for someone who has symptoms or has been diagnosed with a chronic or autoimmune disease.

Maintenance Dosing / Preservation Need: 1-2 teaspoons twice a day
This dose depends on what the individual has determined to be the ideal level of use that maintains the results he or

she sought in the first place. Identifying this level may take some experimentation.

Most people will fall into one of these three categories, and because colostrum is a food, you can't "overdose" on it. Anytime you feel a cold coming on, or your workout was particularly strenuous, or you feel compromised in some manner, you can take more colostrum to accommodate your body's increased need. If illness prevents you from keeping food or fluids down, take small sips of colostrum mixed in water or let a small amount of the powder dissolve under your tongue for a few minutes and then swallow.

As for the timing of when colostrum should be consumed, I recommend one dose upon rising in the morning and before breakfast; the second dose should be taken approximately twelve hours later and at least two hours after the last meal of the day. This ensures that the colostrum bioactives are entering an empty stomach and will remain intact (undigested) as they travel to the small intestine. Ideally, powdered colostrum should be mixed with plain water; food can be consumed twenty to thirty minutes later. There are of course, a few special situations that require different dosing and different timing.

Athletic Performance: 2 Tablespoons twice a day
For professional and amateur athletes, colostrum should be taken prior to a workout and an hour prior to bedtime – on an empty stomach and not combined with a protein source (i.e., protein shake or drink)

Anti-aging: 1-2 Tablespoons twice a day
A larger dose helps supply the growth factors that naturally diminish after puberty. Colostrum provides a natural approach to aging and enhances positive lifestyle choices.

Blood Glucose Balancing or Weight Loss: 1 Tablespoon four times per day

To avoid significant fluctuations in blood sugar levels between meals, include two additional colostrum doses between breakfast/lunch and lunch/dinner. This can help prevent episodes of low blood sugar and make fasting or caloric restriction more tolerable; the leptin in colostrum helps reduce appetite and hunger pangs, if weight loss is the goal.

There are a few situations to be mindful about when taking colostrum, since efficacy is the foremost priority. Avoid taking colostrum with a source of protein (i.e., a protein shake, collagen drink) or with a significant amount of carbohydrates (i.e., a smoothie). If the stomach detects protein or a large volume of food, it will secrete digestive juices which digest and inactivate the colostrum bioactives, especially the growth factors which in turn, break down into amino acids. Therefore, taking colostrum upon rising guarantees an empty stomach, and can be followed by a protein smoothie or breakfast twenty to thirty minutes later. This may take a little pre-planning such as mixing up the colostrum the night before and storing it in the refrigerator.

It may be tempting to add colostrum to hot coffee or tea like a creamer, but this should be avoided. Boiling or very hot water will inactivate colostrum's bioactive components. This is the same rationale behind the use of low-heat drying during the manufacturing process. Mixing colostrum with room temperature or lukewarm water, as well as iced coffee is acceptable, so long as no sugar or milk is added.

I've been asked about whether you can take colostrum while intermittent fasting, and the answer is "yes," and I in fact, recommend it as a best practice. Mix the powdered colostrum in a large volume of plain water and sip at regular intervals throughout the fasting period. Many people have found this to be helpful in getting through the monotony and hunger of intermittent fasting, or fasting in general. I believe it is indeed healthier for the body to receive small but steady amounts of immune bioactives and growth factors during a short-term or long-term water fast.

New or first-time users of colostrum may experience a detox-like event which mimics flu symptoms and may cause temporary mild diarrhea or constipation; this is referred to as Jarisch – Herxheimer reactions, or "herx" for short. As the immunoglobulins, antibodies, lactoferrin, lactoperoxidase, and oligosaccharides destroy gut-based pathogens, the pathogens release toxins which cause the unpleasant symptoms. It's completely normal, and in fact, about one of every five first-time users experience Jarisch – Herxheimer reactions. If symptoms are bothersome, the colostrum dose can be reduced to one-half a teaspoon per day until the body adjusts; then, gradually adjust upwards until the full dose is achieved.

Another consideration for first-time colostrum users is taste, and I'd be remiss if I didn't say colostrum is an acquired taste. It may look creamy and white like milk, but most milk drinkers would not say it tastes or smells like milk. Your senses may be a little offended at first until you get used to it; drinking it cold, with ice cubes, or with a few drops of flavoring may help. Differences in taste, smell, density, and solubility can vary from batch to batch because of the colostrum sourcing (i.e., different cows birthing at different times of the year), the cows' food source (i.e., different food/feed during different seasons), and the ambient humidity levels when the colostrum is processed. If taste or smell are non-starters, then colostrum in capsule form can be substituted. However, powdered colostrum mixed in water is the ideal form because its healing action begins in the mouth, well before a gelatin capsule dissolves further down the G.I. tract.

I also recommend avoiding any probiotic supplements for the first four to six weeks of colostrum supplementation. If the gut lining is leaky, even the "good" bacterial strains in a probiotic supplement will cross over into the bloodstream and illicit an immune reaction. The immune system doesn't differentiate between good and bad bacteria – in the same way it won't recognize an undigested food protein as harmless; it simply identifies a foreign substance invading its realm. Thus, healing a leaky gut prior to introducing any probiotics is critical.

Furthermore, I contend that probiotics need colostrum to colonize in the gut, and without it, the good bacteria strains will simply pass out of the body in a bowel movement. In this regard, colostrum acts like a prebiotic; the growth factors nourish the probiotics and allow them to multiply. The co-mechanism of action is the destruction of bad bacteria by the lactoferrin, lactoperoxidase, and lysozyme that in turn, frees up space for the good bacteria to grow. It is this symbiotic relationship that makes probiotic supplementation without colostrum supplementation a misguided approach to gut health and a waste of money.

Avoiding medications, foods, and other antagonists (*See Chapter 6.*) that irritate the G.I. lining as much as possible is also important to getting a jumpstart on the healing process. If your primary care physician has prescribed any gut-irritating medication(s), check with him or her as to how you can safely cut back or eliminate it completely. Since maintaining the tight junctions of the G.I. lining is an on-going endeavor due to the constant challenges (i.e., life), taking colostrum every day should be viewed as necessary as drinking water every day.

Because health sovereignty relies upon knowledge, the ongoing pursuit of that knowledge is paramount. Health knowledge helps form the basis for good decision-making, and regardless of how one may have grown up, knowledge-empowered adults can choose health for themselves and for their dependent children. Instilling good health habits early in life is a strategic approach to ensure that children will continue on the path of good health throughout life. No one wants a child to needlessly suffer from a chronic disease or a weak immune system, so including colostrum as a dietary foundation becomes an imperative for every parent today.

Infant & Toddler Use: ½ teaspoon twice a day, or as directed by a pediatrician
Parents of newborns, infants, and toddlers should also supplement their child's nutrition with powdered bovine colostrum, especially if the infant is not being breastfed for the first two years. Colostrum from any mammal source is **not** a substitute for mother's breastmilk, but if exclusive or extended breastfeeding is not possible, or if baby is not thriving, bovine colostrum is the best option. If parents object to cow-derived products, goat colostrum may be substituted. Any commercial powdered colostrum supplement should be utilized in conjunction with freshly purified water (not bottled water), filtered apple juice, formula, or age-appropriate foods (i.e., applesauce, yogurt, vegetable puree). Because little ones don't secrete the same harsh stomach acids as adults, they can consume colostrum with food. Upon taking colostrum for the first time, some infants experience a mild sensitivity that may result in changes to stool color or consistency. This is a normal reaction, so begin with ¼ teaspoon for the first few feedings and gradually increase to ½ teaspoon. If symptoms persist, contact your pediatrician for further advice.

I strongly recommend new mothers also supplement with colostrum. It optimizes the immune system to help prevent respiratory infections, re-establishes robust bowel health, and helps metabolize residual fat deposits from pregnancy. Colostrum's positive effect on the gut microbiome improves serotonin production and uptake, thereby helping attenuate post-partum blues. In addition to regular exercise and good nutrition, colostrum helps new mothers get back on their feet so they can take care of their precious little ones, as well as life's busy demands.

Because colostrum helps balance the gut microbiome, it supports the bacteria that synthesize serotonin, dopamine, the B-vitamins, and other important substrates that the body needs to function optimally. Approximately 90-95% of serotonin is produced in the gut, which is not only critical for a good mood and calmness, but is influential in ongoing mental health concerns. And because depression is now viewed as having a neuroinflammatory component,[127,128] any natural substance that can decrease inflammation provides a benefit for mental health. Colostrum – with its anti-inflammatory and gut health-promoting capabilities – may offer a measure of hope for new and/or nursing mothers who may be reluctant to take pharmacologic drugs.

There's no doubt that life today is emotionally stressful for a great many individuals, even those who are normally good at dealing with stress. Often, poor nutritional habits set in or take over when the wherewithal to deal with mental issues becomes overwhelming, and your gut bugs respond accordingly. I highly recommend daily colostrum supplementation for anyone who is going through emotional difficulties and/or stress.

Colostrum offers so many ways to improve health so that we can live longer with less illness, pain and disability, yet colostrum isn't just for humans. Mammalian pets suffer many of the same diseases that humans do, including digestive issues, diabetes, painful joints, dermatitis, and other age-related conditions and so, they can also benefit from bovine colostrum supplementation. Colostrum is also appropriate for preventive use, as it is for humans. Puppies and kittens that have been weaned too early or did not receive their mothers' own colostrum should be fed powdered colostrum mixed with their regular nutritional formula. Research with recently weaned puppies suggests that bovine colostrum can help reduce recurrent diarrhea-causing gastroenteritis and improve vitality in early life.[129] When fed a bovine colostrum-supplemented diet, adult dogs experienced a positive immune response, and their gut microbiome gained more bacterial diversity.[130]

Veterinarians can provide guidance for your pet's specific need, which are predicated on these general guidelines:

Mammalian Pet Use: twice daily based on weight
   1 – 10 pounds: ½ teaspoon
   10 – 40 pounds: 1 teaspoon
   40 – 100 pounds: 2 teaspoons

Very large animals, such as horses, are typically fed veterinary-grade bovine colostrum; this type of colostrum does not meet the high immunoglobulin standard of human-grade bovine colostrum. It would be cost-prohibitive to feed horses the necessary quantity of human-grade colostrum.

Colostrum's growth factors make it ideal for topical skin care, including minor wounds, and can be used for both people and animals. It may also be used as a cosmeceutical for anti-aging skin care. Whenever colostrum is utilized topically, it should be complemented with oral supplementation for maximum benefit.

Minor Wound Care Use: once or twice daily
For the topical healing of minor burns, abrasions, and cuts, clean the wound thoroughly; pat dry with a clean cloth and apply a light dusting of powdered colostrum with a sterile cotton ball before bandaging. Repeat every time the dressing is changed.

Cosmeceutical Use / Anti-Wrinkle Cream: once daily at bedtime
Place a normal amount of your favorite overnight moisturizer in the palm of your hand and add 1 teaspoon of powdered colostrum; combine thoroughly and apply to face and/or

neck as you normally would. Alternatively, mix ½ teaspoon powdered colostrum with enough purified water, extra virgin olive oil, or coconut oil to easily apply around the eyes. Cleanse your face in the morning.

Cosmeceutical Use / Facial Mask: as often as desired

Mix 1-2 Tablespoons of powdered colostrum with enough purified water to make a thick paste; apply evenly to face and/or neck and allow paste to dry; rinse with cool water and pat dry.

Vaginal Well-being: once daily, or as needed

Mix 1-2 teaspoons of colostrum into 4-6 ounces of sterile water; pour into a vaginal douche bag. Gently squeeze the solution into the vagina and allow to drain normally. Be sure to thoroughly clean the douche bag between uses.

Health sovereignty is not a health fad and neither is bovine colostrum. There's a fundamental reason that colostrum is our first food – the first food of life. It eases the pain and inflammation as we are literally squished and squeezed through the birth canal, and as we enter a world of microbes – some friend, some foe – it jumpstarts the immune system that we come to rely upon for a lifetime. The intimate and loving act of breastfeeding helps bond mother and child, as it imparts nourishment and health. A solid foundation is more important now than ever before and as the world becomes a smaller place with its well-traveled pathogens, immune resilience is the key to our survival. Once we are weaned from our mothers' breasts, supplemental bovine colostrum provides the immune bioactives and growth factors necessary to sustain good health and maintain physical and mental homeostasis.

TENETS TO LIVE BY

Nutrition	• Organic, nutrient-dense, minimally processed foods • Antioxidant-rich, fresh vegetables and fruits • Sustainably raised meats • Low sugar • High-fiber • Healthy fats • Clean drinking water
Physical Activity	• Daily activity & minimal sitting • 150 minutes of structured exercise weekly • Recreational (fun) activity
Sleep	• 7-8 hours high-quality sleep nightly
Emotional Stress	• Regular stress management activities • Professional therapy, if necessary
Mindset	• Openness to new ideas & experiences • Self-acceptance & commitment to improvement • Positive attitude • Regular mental & social engagement • Honesty & civility • Expression of gratitude & kindness

Eat to live, not live to eat.
Socrates

CHAPTER 12

Aging Well: Live Longer. Feel Better. And Look Great Doing It.

I can talk about health sovereignty until I'm blue in the face – and sometimes, I think I glimpse a cerulean hue when I look in the mirror at the end of the day. At any given moment, we're all at very different places in our lives. We may be young and healthy and can't imagine becoming anything like our parents or grandparents…in poor health, hunched over with wrinkled skin and thinning, greying hair, and ten or more extra pounds around the middle. Or we may already see those changes happening gradually with each passing decade, or perhaps full-throttle as if both ends of the candle are furiously burning with no fire extinguisher in sight. It's difficult to convince young people that what they do now will affect them ten, twenty, or thirty years down the road; feeling good in the moment overrides the ability to forecast or even imagine how future health will impact one's quality of life. But, by the time one reaches the fourth or fifth decade, the willingness to listen begins to grow stronger. The sounds we hear are more than just minor aches and pains or creaky joints. It's also the sound of wallets opening…offering up big bucks to buy the latest and greatest anti-aging solution.

Two things are certain when it comes to growing older: No one wants to *feel* old, and no one wants to *look* old. The latter may be true more so and for far more people because

Western societies place such a high value on maintaining a youthful appearance. And while today, there are surgical procedures, chemical applications, diet plans, energy concoctions, and anti-aging self-help books, time continues in a singular direction. So too, does your internal odometer which reflects your body's state of wear and tear caused by inflammation and oxidative stress. So, ask yourself: *Does my internal odometer reflect city miles [highly inflammatory/lots of oxidative stress] or highway miles [less inflammatory/less oxidative stress]?* You may have been born with great genes, but poor lifestyle kept the good genes in the "off" position, or worse yet, turned on the bad genes. Although the calendar says you're fifty, you may feel ten years older and your appearance prompts the grocery store clerk to give you the senior (65+) discount without asking.

The key to aging well is to maintain good health for as long as possible (i.e., healthspan), thereby staving off any extreme disability or serious illness until the very end of life. I've talked about how bovine colostrum supplementation can assist in this regard, as it helps counterbalance the body's natural tapering off of growth hormone and insulin-like growth factor-1 (IGF-1) production following puberty. Some thirty years ago, researchers generated quite a buzz about synthetic human growth hormone being the new Fountain of Youth for its ability to retard the decrease in lean body mass, slow the increase in adipose tissue, and decelerate the thinning of the skin that occurs with normal aging.[131,132] Additional purported – and masterfully marketed – benefits included improvements to one's stamina and energy levels, metabolism, weight loss, insulin sensitivity, bone density, flexibility, skin elasticity, memory, sleep, mood, immunity, wound healing, libido, and sexual performance. A great body, a great mind, and great sex... Who wouldn't want any or all of these amazing results? Patients flocked to their doctors, hoping to persuade them to prescribe growth hormone for off-label use as a youth-restoring treatment.

The first synthetic version of growth hormone had been developed and approved in 1985 for treating short stature and poor growth in children; limited use in adults has been approved since then but not for anti-aging or athletic use. In the early 1990s, researchers found that longer-term administration of the synthetic hormone could induce serious side effects in elderly men, such as carpal tunnel syndrome and gynecomastia, which generally reversed if patients stopped taking it; however, the benefits also reversed.[133] Subsequent research identified additional side effects including muscle and joint pain; soft tissue swelling; elevated fasting blood glucose levels; increased type 2 diabetes risk; elevated cholesterol levels; and no improvement in functional ability.[134,135] Another serious concern was that taking an isolated hormone could potentially promote cancer cells to grow and multiply. So, what initially appeared to be a highly prized discovery was instead fraught with dangerous side effects. Still, the allure of turning back the odometer and reclaiming one's youth was a powerful motivator for patients. For medical providers, the allure of making a lot of money with minimal effort was extremely appealing and soon, a bevy of anti-aging clinics and Internet pharmacies popped up touting growth hormone to anyone willing to pay.

The benefits of synthetic growth hormone and also of endogenous growth hormone are in fact, due to the action of IGF-1 – something that is certainly less well-known by the general public and even by many medical professionals. The human pituitary gland secretes growth hormone during the day, which then travels to the liver and stimulates the liver to produce IGF-1. With a similar molecular structure and action to that of insulin, IGF-1 plays a significant role in cell division and cell growth, and it affects nearly every tissue in the body. In essence, IGF-1 is the "real" growth hormone, yet it too, declines with advancing age. So, from the Fountain of Youth perspective, bovine colostrum is a safe, all-natural, and economical anti-aging supplement.

Throughout this book, I've primarily focused on taking colostrum internally because of its significant impact on gut and immune health, yet colostrum's anti-aging benefits are not limited to the "inside skin," or the lining of the G.I. tract. Certainly, it's true that when people are healthier on the inside, they look better on the outside; their skin has a noticeable glow, looks hydrated, and has a supple texture. A state of immunocompromise often has people looking years older than their chronological age, so in addition to supplementing daily with colostrum, topical application presents a unique opportunity for its aesthetic potential.

Furthermore, there is a connection between the "inside skin" and the "outside skin" in terms of their function; both are considered barrier organs and are the first lines of immune defense for the human body. They each host a distinct yet related microbiome, and they are comprised of similar features, including thin layers of cells, tight junctions between cells, cells that send messages to the immune system (dendritic cells), and cells that selectively control the absorption of nutrients. The communication between the two microbiomes – called the gut-skin axis – signifies the important role that bacteria in the gut microbiome play in skin health and appearance.[136,137] Beneficial gut bacteria manufacture the neurotransmitters that facilitate protective biological reactions which are hormone sensitive. In other words, outside skin that looks and feels healthy and is without eruptions is dependent on a healthy gut microbiome and a strong, non-porous G.I. lining.

Leaky gut and gut dysbiosis don't just lead to autoimmune conditions affecting tissues and organs within the body, but also to autoimmune skin conditions such as eczema, psoriasis, rosacea, scleroderma, systemic lupus erythematosus, atopic dermatitis, and acne vulgaris. These inflammatory skin conditions result from the immune system attacking the cells that comprise the various layers of skin. It is quite possible that some individuals exhibit skin symptoms before physically experiencing a gut problem. In this case, the skin is sort of like a mirror as to what is happening in the gut.[138] This is why good nutrition and colostrum early in life are important to gut health that translates into beautiful skin throughout life (assuming you don't over-indulge in sun-worshipping and refrain from smoking).

Likewise, the skin microbiome has the capacity to produce a variety of hormones, neurotransmitters, and vitamin D that in turn, influence whole-body health. Some research suggests that the skin microbiome may contribute to neurotransmitter production that affects our emotions.[139] So, just like the nutrition we obtain through food and supplements affects microbial diversity in the gut and overall physical and mental health, the "nutrition" we expose our skin microbiome to affects microbial diversity and contributes to health of the whole body, and quite possibly emotional well-being. As an interface to all that makes us human and second in size to the G.I. lining, the skin serves as a barrier to environmental insults – the "nutrition" we expose it to – such as air pollution, UV rays, and topical chemical exposure. Healthy skin cells of the epidermis layer (the outermost skin layer) produce superoxide dismutase (SOD), an antioxidant enzyme that helps neutralize free radicals, particularly those created by UV exposure. Therefore, a compromised epidermis can lead to skin cell damage, skin cancer, and contribute to the undesirable signs of skin aging. And, let's not forget that the outside skin is second only to the liver as a detoxification organ for the entire body.

Indulge me as I make a brief mention of milk baths (an

early form of skin nutrition) as a beauty ritual dating back to the Ancient Egyptians. Allegedly, Queen Cleopatra regularly bathed in donkey milk to preserve her legendary beauty and fair skin, and there may actually be some validity to this story – or at least a rationale behind its use. The growth factors in raw dairy milk (to a lesser extent than in raw colostrum), as well as the vitamins and minerals would have improved aging of the skin and remediated damage caused by sun exposure and a dry climate. As the name implies, skin growth factors encourage skin cells to accelerate their capacity for repair and regeneration, thereby more quickly replacing old, dead skin cells with new ones for a more radiant appearance. This ritual – reportedly requiring the milk of 7,000 donkeys – would be a tremendous undertaking for anyone of normal means, but targeted topical colostrum application is definitely more realistic today.

Growth factors with the most significant impact for anti-aging include insulin-like growth factor-1 (IGF-1), transforming growth factors (TGF-α and TGF-β), epidermal/epithelial growth factor (EGF), fibroblast growth factor (FGF), and platelet-derived growth factor (PDGF). Bovine colostrum contains these in relative abundance and as such, shows promise for skin damage caused by chemical burns, lacerations, puncture wounds, as well as normal and accelerated photoaging. Applying colostrum to the face – either directly or as an ingredient in a commercial facial cream – has sparked great interest in recent years for its potential as a natural anti-aging remedy. The growing trend, particularly as more clinical research is done, will likely position bovine colostrum as either a "cosmeceutical" or "dermaceutical."

But wait…there's more…more compelling data about colostrum's benefit to skin health, chromosome (DNA) longevity, and aging in general. Telomere attrition, or shortening, is thought to be one of several mechanisms that contributes to the development of age-related diseases and the outward signs of skin aging. Once we make our entrance into the world, our cellular time in human form becomes finite. The presence – and absence – of the telomerase enzyme influences how many times the cell (and all its critical DNA) can successfully divide before it ultimately runs out of dividing capability. Telomerase mediates the repair of the telomeres (end caps of the chromosomes, like shoelace end caps), and without telomerase, the chromosomes become a tiny bit shorter until one day, that cell is unable to divide at all. Two significant consequences of telomere shortening are the inability of body tissues to regenerate themselves and poor immune response, or immunocompromise.

The erosion, or fraying, of the telomeres is one way to quantify the aging process. Some people age more quickly than others (i.e., more erosion), and their telomeres undergo accelerated shortening. Shorter telomeres, and thus, accelerated biological aging, is associated with telomerase deficiency, and shorter telomeres correlate with increased disease risk.[140] Analyzing a person's telomere length or the telomere attrition rate can be useful predictors of who might develop certain diseases such as cardiovascular disease, type 2 diabetes, and certain types of cancer.[141,142,143] Since the telomeres' lengths within any given cell may vary, the shortest telomeres are a predictor of risk, not the average length of all the telomeres in the cell. In other words, the presence of just one or a few shortened telomeres – in the absence of telomerase – can, in turn, induce DNA damage or cell death. This is not the case with every cell type, but it does give us reason to be concerned, as it can lead to early onset of disease.

Measuring telomere length may be a useful tool to predict which individuals may later develop certain diseases, especially if they are currently asymptomatic. It would be like looking into a crystal ball but knowing that one's health fate isn't necessarily sealed and that by making positive changes, the outcome can be completely different. Life's behavior stressors (i.e., poor diet, physical inactivity, tobacco use, chemical exposure, alcohol/substance abuse) as well as psychological stress and the stress of chronic disease itself can increase telomere attrition rate in adults. The good news is that all of these stressors can be minimized or eliminated by changing how you choose to live your life going forward.

The sad news is, however, that childhood trauma (i.e., exposure to stress, neglect, violence, poor nutrition/malnutrition) can shorten telomeres in children. Seminal research involving children in Romanian orphanages showed that the more time spent living in an orphanage the shorter their telomeres, and many children had smaller brains, reduced brain activity, lower IQs, stunted physical growth, and difficulty forming lasting relationships.[144] War, famine, disease (i.e., HIV/AIDS, Ebola, and now SARS-CoV-2), and socioeconomic inequality have and will continue to create childhood trauma, but we shouldn't forget about bad parenting, which also creates emotional scars. Physical or verbal abuse, neglect, abandonment via divorce, lack of mothering, and stress sensitivity can impact telomere length, and the effects flow into adulthood. These include poor health behaviors (i.e., eating disorders, alcoholism, substance abuse, other addictions) and dysfunctional personal relationships.

Telomere attrition in children can be ameliorated to some degree, but it's the adults who must take responsibility and action for making these kids whole again. Early intervention to address a child's adverse situation, minimize the stressors, and remedy the emotional issues can help lessen the rate of telomere shortening. If you have experienced any type of childhood trauma that affects your current behavior and/or relationships, it's well worth the effort to protect your telomeres from degrading further or faster. Another very good reason to be telomere-cognizant is if you are a woman who wants to have a baby (or even a grandchild). A woman with short telomeres in her eggs – resulting from her own childhood trauma – can transmit short telomeres to her child. Or, if she experiences stress or poor health during pregnancy, she can also transmit these short (or shorter) telomeres to her child. Her offspring could in turn, do the same.

The dramatic way in which trauma can affect children is one of the reasons I advocate for early and extended breastfeeding. Far from being a proven "telomere reset," I do think that a nursing mother can impart the "gift of health" to her newborn and perhaps, prevent accelerated telomere shortening in both herself and her child. This bonding time also provides psychological benefits for both mother and child that may help reduce the effect of life's stressors. In adults, daily bovine colostrum supplementation combined with healthy lifestyle behaviors may offer a potential defense against telomere shortening as well.

Currently, telomere analysis is not part of routine medical screenings due to the cost. A few companies sell an at-home blood sample collection kit and genetic testing with a blood draw that can be ordered by physicians for the purpose of determining one's cellular age versus chronological age. As the cost of this technology undoubtedly will go down in the near future, knowing your telomere attrition rate will be as common as knowing your cholesterol levels. But until that time, we can take action to slow, maintain, or reverse telomere loss through lifestyle and dietary interventions – the goal of which is to increase telomerase activity in the cells. Keep in mind that most cells in the body contain little to no telomerase, so the ability to "anti-age" is probably limited. Researchers are just now beginning to understand the implications of telomeres, yet, there's never a downside to an all-around healthy (and telomere-friendly) lifestyle that minimizes inflammation and oxidative stress. This should include regular exercise, stress management, sufficient sleep, mindfulness, and an omega-3-rich, antioxidant-rich diet.[145] Periodic telomere analysis allows patients and physicians to track the effect of positive lifestyle changes on biological aging over time.

Although the evidence is scant, raw, unprocessed bovine colostrum is purported to contain the telomerase enzyme, and I am inclined to believe that may be true. If not, *something* in colostrum slows telomere attrition, and that may in part, be responsible for the anti-aging effects we're observing. This would further support its use as both a nutritional supplement and as a topical application for skin rejuvenation. A recent *in vitro* study showed that when colostrum was added to human fibroblast cells (collagen-producing cells within connective tissue), the fibroblasts replicated themselves at a higher rate and their telomeres shortened at a slower rate than without colostrum.[146] Furthermore, when hydrogen peroxide (H_2O_2) was added to the cells to induce oxidative stress, telomere shortening was accelerated, but when H_2O_2 and colostrum were added together, the telomeres did not shorten within the observed time period of eight weeks. The mechanism of action is unclear, but certainly would make for some interesting research in the future.

When it comes to skin health and looking younger, reducing telomere erosion is not the only potential benefit of topically applied colostrum. The growth factors discussed previously, as well as cytokines, are known to promote collagen synthesis.[147,148] Fine lines and wrinkles are essentially "wounds," and research in both humans and other mammals has demonstrated colostrum's ability to promote more rapid wound healing.[149,150] Depending on the type of wound – superficial or deep – colostrum powder can be applied directly to the uncovered wound or in combination with a sterile dressing. For fine lines and wrinkles, powdered colostrum should be made into a thin paste using purified water and applied evenly (*Refer to Chapter 11 for a DIY recipe*).

Another type of "wound" is vulvovaginal atrophy, which occurs when a woman's estrogen levels decline significantly during and after menopause. Approximately fifty percent of postmenopausal women experience thinning of the skin-like tissue of the vulva and vagina, which often leads to vaginal dryness, irritation, painful intercourse, bleeding, urinary frequency, urgency, and incontinence, all of which may contribute to decreased libido. Vulvovaginal atrophy is typically treated with vaginal lubricants and/or estrogen replacement therapy, yet there is growing interest in using bovine colostrum as a vaginal gel ingredient to help remediate vaginal dryness, strengthen vaginal tissue, and improve other unpleasant symptoms.[151,152] From an anti-aging and sexual health perspective, this type of product has shown to increase women's overall quality of life as well as sexual satisfaction.[153]

With the realization that women's sexual health and sexual satisfaction are important issues, a reckoning is upon us. The use of bovine colostrum as a potential aid has become more than simply anecdotal...it's now ripe for scientific research, and I expect it to play a role in the arena of natural vaginal rejuvenation. And let's not forget that fulfilling sexual relationships are important for both men and women at any age, in spite of natural hormonal changes throughout life. Remaining active, healthy, and free from sexual impairment are beneficial to any couple – whether you've been together for five, twenty-five, or fifty years. Looking good (or great) naked is icing on the cake.

And as long as I'm on the topic of cake...let's discuss oxidation. The biological processes of digesting and metabolising the nutrients in food yields metabolic waste by-products called reactive oxygen species (ROS), including free radicals, peroxides, lipid peroxides, and heavy metals. A youthful body can handle recycling of ROS relatively well, but with advancing age, an accumulation of ROS causes oxidative stress in the tissues and fuels rapid aging. Certainly, there are other good and poor lifestyle habits (strenuous exercise, smoking) that create ROS, but the one life activity everyone partakes in is eating. Well-regarded animal research by Clive Maine McCay, Ph.D. in the 1930s showed that calorie-restricted, but not malnourished rats lived substantially longer than rats allowed to eat without restriction.[154] Dr. McCay's research helped unite the various academic fields contributing to the study of old age and the aging process (gerontology). Today, the consensus for non-obese individuals is that well-nourished calorie restriction (i.e., no empty, but fewer calories) decreases biomarkers of aging, promotes metabolic health, and does not adversely affect quality of life.[155]

I believe that bovine colostrum should be the foundational supplement for any well-nourished calorie restricted eating plan because among its diverse bioactives and nutrients, colostrum contains glutathione and its building blocks cystine, glycine, and glutamic acid in abundance.[156] Often referred to as the "mother of all antioxidants," glutathione functions to clean up the ROS, thereby preventing cellular, DNA, and mitochondrial damage. Although glutathione itself is not absorbed in the intestines, its precursors are and from there, contribute to glutathione production throughout the body. Ingesting bovine colostrum daily helps to ensure an ample supply of glutathione to combat ROS and the effects of aging, but it's not a substitute for healthy eating.

Sometimes, even "healthy eating" leads to weight gain as we get older, and unhealthy eating just gets us there quicker. The finely-tuned twenty-year-old machine of yesteryear has lost some (or a lot) of its metabolic efficiency, and the extra calories are stored for that proverbial rainy-day adipose fund that is never utilized. Colostrum's leptin can help decrease appetite, thus making weight loss easier. And when taken between meals, colostrum helps modulate blood glucose levels so you're less inclined to experience low blood sugar (hypoglycemia) and snack or overeat between meals. Individuals who fast regularly for weight control or detox – whether intermittent, once a week, or a few days at a time – have found colostrum quite useful in maintaining the fast without feeling overly hungry or hangry. When regular exercise, and particularly strength training, is added to your weight loss strategy, colostrum helps build lean muscle tissue which in turn, burns more stored calories from the adipose fund.

Maybe you can live with the extra pounds or the wrinkles...you've convinced yourself that they're signs of a more mature person. But then the pain of creaky joints, and you begin feeling like you're getting "old." Whether you experience minor muscle aches and joint pain from exercise or chronic pain from the lack of exercise and/or from disease or injury, daily supplementation with bovine colostrum can help attenuate pain by reducing inflammation. Colostrum's anti-inflammatory cytokines are a natural way to reduce inflamed tissue and help the immune system return to homeostasis. Achieving resiliency should be the goal, not causing additional tissue damage by using over-the-counter and prescription pain medications. And when you're not in pain, everything else is much easier. Aging well is easier.

Other hypothesized mechanisms of human aging in addition to telomere erosion, include cellular senescence (cell death), stem cell exhaustion, mitochondrial dysfunction, genomic instability, epigenetic changes, altered intercellular

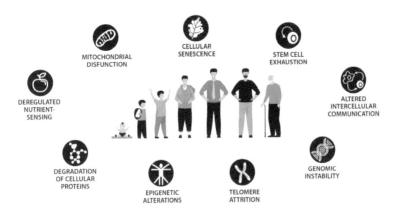

Figure 6: Multifactorial Causes of Aging

communication, deregulated nutrient sensing, and the inappropriate folding and/or degradation of cellular proteins (*See Figure 6*). Whew! That's a whole lot that could possibly go wrong, and it makes us realize just how complicated and simultaneously amazing the human body really is. The field of gerontology guides us towards a greater understanding of human aging and of maximizing healthspan for the purpose of living life to our fullest potential. Hippocrates said, "*Health is the greatest of human blessings,*" to which I add, "*Aging well is a gift to oneself.*" Once you learn, practice, and exert mastery over the minute-by-minute biological processes that influence your body and mind, you've gifted yourself. Colostrum provides the foundation to get started, and no matter where you are on the age spectrum, today is the perfect day to begin aging well.

CONCLUSION
Is Anyone Listening Now?

When all is said and read, I hope I've made a compelling argument for health sovereignty and bovine colostrum supplementation to promote immune resiliency, healthspan, and quality of life. I began by telling you that the Centers for Disease Control and Prevention (CDC) records six in ten American adults as having a chronic disease and four in ten having two or more chronic diseases,[157] and that nearly every American will die of an autoimmune disease. Our current reality is shameful, particularly when we know how to prevent or delay disease onset with better lifestyle and nutrition habits.

The year 2020 witnessed a highly infectious virus inflict even greater suffering and premature death on individuals with existing chronic diseases and plague even the strongest bodies with lingering symptoms. Half way into 2021, at the time of this writing, we are still in the grip of a mutating virus. When the COVID-19 pandemic eventually comes to an "end," we may be dealing with it similarly to the seasonal flu – still deadly in its own right. One thing I'm certain of is that other pandemics will undoubtedly follow. It's my sincere hope that we'll be better prepared the next time. To be forewarned is to be forearmed.

So much of human health is owed to the health of the immune system. For Kaye and many like her, they learned the hard way – through no fault of their own. And even though thymus radiation is no longer an accepted medical treatment, it was the medical truth as was currently known and understood at the time. Today, it gives us pause to think about whether current therapies for various conditions may be doing patients more harm than good. Is the cure worse than the disease? Are the big gun antibiotics destroying the gut microbiome and leaving us defenseless against the next little bug that comes from Grandma's potato salad? Or are the opioids prescribed for an old high school injury damaging the gut lining and allowing undigested food proteins, pathogens, and environmental toxins free access to the body where they precipitate an over-reaction, creating a downward spiral towards autoimmunity?

What we eat, drink, and otherwise put into our bodies entails personal choice. These are some of the big issues we need to think about if we are to have a realistic chance of avoiding premature aging and an untimely death. And it goes without saying that no one wants unnecessary physical or mental suffering, especially years or decades of pain, or even what we witnessed in COVID-19 patients. Quality of life is integral to human existence, and we are acutely aware of this now more than perhaps any other point in time.

I hope these pages have not only introduced you to the health benefits of bovine colostrum, but also inspired you to make changes in your daily life that will guide you towards improved immune resiliency and overall health and well-being. I appreciate each and every one of you for taking this journey with me, as it has been my life's work ever since that life-altering day when Kaye asked me to help her die. My relationship with Kaye – albeit much too short – taught me just how precious life is and how truly blessed one is to have found his or her soulmate. Once this blessing is realized – perhaps by the grace of God – you attain completeness. And as I found myself willing to go to the ends of the earth to make Kaye whole again, I found my own path forward – to rediscover a long forgotten natural remedy and reintroduce it to people in need of a "healing miracle."

Additionally, I hope that whether you're a healthcare professional, a mother-to-be, or a friend of someone who is expecting that you now understand the importance of breastfeeding, if you did not already. I humbly ask you to advocate for breastfeeding and the social issues it entails, whether you are a mother or not. The saying, *breast is best* firmly resonates within concept of immune resiliency. Mother Nature intended for mammalian offspring to receive the immune-supporting and growth-enhancing bioactives in both colostrum and milk to drive a species' survival. The science may be catching up to prove their importance for thriving, not simply surviving in humans. Kaye survived without her mother's colostrum, but she thrived afterwards with bovine colostrum.

And speaking of the science, colostrum's wide range of potential health benefits has stirred even greater interest for research and clinical trials. The number of completed and recruiting clinical trials registered with the National Institutes of Health (NIH) is at an all-time high.[158] As of the end of 2020, clinical trials of bovine colostrum or its bioactives involved pre-term infant health, athletic performance, alcoholic hepatitis, non-alcoholic fatty liver disease, HIV, vulvovaginal atrophy, acute lymphoblastic leukemia, multiple organ dysfunction syndrome, diabetes, severe acute malnutrition, influenza, diarrhea, and various infections. (*See Appendix C for a list of NIH-sponsored trials.*) With exciting research in progress and on the horizon, the future of the colostrum industry looks bright.

My journey to rediscover colostrum has had its fair share of ups and downs, successes and failures, celebrations and frustrations, but all in all, it's this labor of love that keeps me strong. I've had the pleasure of meeting people from around the world who became colostrum advocates either through personal experience or professional experience – individuals and patients who recovered their health by taking bovine colostrum and choosing healthy habits. I've had the good fortune to work with scientists in various fields who've committed themselves to understanding the healing potential of bovine colostrum and to advancing its use as a foundational nutritional supplement. I have a dedicated and energetic team who is (almost) as passionate about colostrum as I am and together, we work towards the shared goal of educating consumers through my non-profit organization, the Vibrant Life Institute (VibrantLifeInstitute.org). Our wish for you is optimal health.

So, it is with gratitude I thank God for my life, my time with Kaye, and all of you. I have shared what I know, and now I humbly ask the same of you – to share the gift of health... the healing miracle of colostrum.

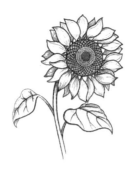

Epilogue

My Dearest Kaye:

Although you are no longer with us, I feel you near to me – often. Before our journey together began, I was myself on a journey – a spiritual journey to find peace and wholeness. Like many who experience the horrors of war, I was not whole for a very long time. The day we met was transformational for me and I still find it inexplicable, except to put my faith in God that it was all part of His plan.

Under my breath, and without realizing, I uttered, "There she is... " You were the most beautiful woman I'd ever seen. Within moments, as if God grabbed me by the collar, pried me out of my seat, and dragged me towards you, I was sitting by your side. "I don't know why but I have to tell you a story about why I'm here. It's just bubbling out of me. I see you in my mind and my heart. I've known you forever. I see you dancing with me. You're wearing an off-white dress, with a diagonal hem cut on the bias. There's a big band playing and I'm so in love with you."

You must have thought I was crazy, intoxicated, arrogant, cruel, or some of each. Your beet-red face certainly couldn't hide your lividity. "Who put you up to this? How could you possibly know this? There's only two people in the world that know I've been dreaming about this my whole life... ever since I was a little girl. I had these vivid dreams about dancing under Japanese lanterns, and I hear the music."

"I know. That's me you're dancing with."

"That couldn't be! My brother and my mother are the only people who know about this. They must have put you up to this. This is a practical joke, isn't it?"

"No, I'm very serious. I don't know your brother or your mother. I'm going to prove something to you, but you'll have to come out to my car. Come out to my car... please... and I'll play you the music you've been hearing in your mind and your heart."

I thank God you indulged me that day, and seeing the tears stream down your face when you heard Frank Sinatra serenading us from my 8-track player, I felt my transformation begin.

Yours in eternal gratitude,
Douglas

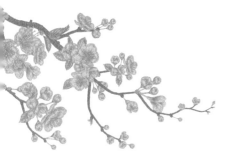

IN APPRECIATION

It's Been A Decades-Long Group Effort
Thank you...

Andrew Keech, Ph.D.
...for your dedication to quality and excellence. Your world-renown knowledge of colostrum peptides and your colostrum processing expertise has propelled the supplement industry towards what it is today.

Donald R. Henderson, M.D., M.P.H.
...for your open and inquisitive mind. I am grateful for the support you offered Kaye and me as we struggled to get our message about colostrum out to as many people as we could. You were truly one of the original modern-day colostrum advocates.

Graeme Clegg
...for your friendship. You are a genuine inspiration for anyone starting a business from humble means; your sheep-shearing days are a testament to exquisite physical fitness and form. You personify "aging well," and I can only hope to have half your energy and vitality as an octogenarian.

Michail Borissenko, M.S.
...for the Institute of Colostrum Research. Your scientific study of colostrum contributed a wealth of knowledge towards the collective understanding of colostrum's benefits.

Tom White, Ph. C.
...for embodying my goal for all medical practitioners. Your insistence on bovine colostrum for every one of your patients is a credit to your caring nature, and your inflammatory biomarker testing is a credit to colostrum's success. I supplied product, and you gave me scientific evidence to share – an invaluable gift.

Mark J. Tager, M.D.
...for your medical perspective and guidance. It isn't always what I've wanted to hear, but once it sinks in, I know you're (probably) right.

The art of healing comes from nature, not from the physician. Therefore the physician must start from nature, with an open mind.

Paracelsus

Appendix A:
Bioactive Components in Bovine Colostrum

Much of the knowledge related to colostrum's bioactive components was gained through veterinary research and the dairy industry as it relates to successful calving. Kaye and I compiled this list from our exhaustive literature search at the University of Utah's medical library in the 1990s. As more research became available through PubMed, we added to the list. It's important to note that the presence and concentrations of specific components can be influenced by geographical location of the herd, maternal lineage, dietary composition, and exposure to humans (as related to specific antibodies produced). Many of these substances are present in both colostrum and milk, at varying quantities.

Immunoglobulins
IgA (serum IgA)
sIgA (secretory IgA)
IgD
IgEbf (IgE binding factor)
IgG
IgM
Anti-bacterial Antibodies
Bacillus cereus – food poisoning
Streptococcus pyogenes – strep throat and other strep diseases, septicemia
Streptococcus agalactiae – septicemia and meningitis in newborns (vaginal birth)
Streptococcus pneumoniae – pneumonia, ear infections, bacterial meningitis
Streptococcus mutans – periodontal disease, tooth decay, endocarditis, arteriosclerosis

Staphylococcus epidermidis – biofilms on surgical implants and catheters

Staphylococcus aureus – food poisoning, atopic dermatitis, respiratory disease, pneumonia, meningitis, osteomyelitis, endocarditis, toxic shock syndrome, bacteremia, and sepsis

Listeria monocytogenes – listeriosis (food poisoning), meningitis in newborns (vaginal birth)

Yersinia enterocolitica – food poisoning, yersiniosis (bloody diarrhea and fever), septicemia

Escherichia coli – cholecystitis, bacteremia, cholangitis, urinary tract infections, traveler's diarrhea, meningitis, and pneumonia

Escherichia coli O157:H7 – enterohemorrhagic strain of E. coli that can lead to kidney failure

Haemophilus influenzae – pneumonia and acute bacterial meningitis

Campylobacter jejuni – food poisoning

Helicobacter pylori – peptic ulcers

Salmonella enteritidis – food poisoning

Salmonella typhimurium – salmonellosis, enteric fevers (typhoid and paratyphoid)

Klebsiella pneumoniae – pneumonia, meningitis, liver abscesses, endophthalimitis

Propionibacterium acnes – acne

Vibrio cholerae – cholera

Anti-viral Antibodies

Adenovirus – upper respiratory tract infections in children; a variety of adult infections including respiratory disease, conjunctivitis, and gastroenteritis

Alphavirus – arthritis, encephalitis, rashes and fever; includes Sindbis virus and Semliki Forest virus.

Dengue virus – mosquito-borne Dengue fever

Echovirus – febrile illness common in children; the most common cause of aseptic meningitis.

Epstein-Barr & Human Herpes Virus-6 – chronic fatigue syndrome

Enterovirus 71 – hand, foot and mouth disease and other serious neurological diseases

Hantavirus – hemorrhagic fever with renal syndrome and hantavirus pulmonary disease.

Hepatitis C virus – hepatitis C

Herpes viruses – herpes

HIV-1 – HIV

Human Papilloma virus – cervical and other sexually-transmitted cancers

Influenza – seasonal flu

Japanese encephalitis – mosquito-borne viral infection causing encephalitis

Measles virus – measles and associated respiratory complications

Polio virus – poliomyelitis (polio)

Respiratory syncytial virus – lower respiratory tract infections during infancy and childhood

Rotavirus – infectious, often fatal diarrhea among young children worldwide

St. Louis virus – mosquito-borne viral infection causing encephalitis

West Nile virus – mosquito-borne virus encephalitis or meningitis

Yellow fever virus – mosquito-borne virus causing acute hemorrhagic disease that may cause liver damage

Anti-fungal Antibodies

Candida albicans – opportunistic oral (thrush) and genital (vaginal yeast) infections

Complement (C3)

Lactoferrin (lactotransferrin)

Lactoferricin

Lactoperoxidase

Lysozyme
Oligosaccharides
    Fucose
    Galactose
    Glucose
    Mannose
    N-acetyl-galactosamine
    N-acetyl-glucosamine
    N-acetyl-neuraminic acid
    Xylose
Proline-rich Polypeptides (PRPs, colostrinin)
Cytokines
    Chemokines
    CXCL 1-7 (CXC chemokine ligands)
    CXCL 8
    Eotaxin
    GRO-alpha (growth related protein alpha)
Interferons
    Interferon-γ (IFNγ)
    P-10 (interferon-γ inducible protein)
    MCP-1 (monocyte chemotactic protein)
    MIG (monokine induced by interferon-γ)
    RANTES (Regulated upon Activation, Normal T cell
        Expressed and Secreted)
Lymphokines
Interleukins
    Interleukin 1β (IL-1β)
    Interleukin 2 (IL-2)
    Interleukin 4 (IL-4)
    Interleukin 5 (IL-5)
    Interleukin 6 (IL-6)
    Interleukin 8 (IL-8)
    Interleukin 10 (IL-10)
    Interleukin 12 (IL-12)
    Interleukin 13 (IL-13)

Interleukin 16 (IL-16)
Interleukin 18 (IL-18)
Tumor necrosis factors (TNF)
TNF-α
TNF-α receptors
Osteopontin
Osteoprotegerin

Protease Inhibitors
α2-macroglobulin
α2-antiplasmin
Antithrombin III
C1-inhibitor
Chymotrypsin inhibitor
Elastase inhibitor
Inter-α-trypsin inhibitor
Trypsin inhibitor (α1-antitrypsin)

Casein Peptides
κ-caseino glycomacropeptide
κ-caseinoglycopeptide

Hemopexin
Haptoglobin
Thrombospondin
Milk Globule Membrane Proteins
Mucin 1 (MUC1)
BAMP (Bovine Associated Mucoprotein)
Lactadherin
Adipophilin
Butyrophilin
CD36 (fatty acid translocase)

α2-macroglobulin
β2-microglobulin (thymotaxin, lactollin)
Lipocalins
β-lactoglobulin
Fatty acid binding protein
Clusterin (Apolipoprotein J)

Casein
    α-casein
    β-casein
    κ-casein
Orosomucoids (α1-acid glycoprotein)
Folate-binding protein
α-lactalbumin
Multimeric α-lactalbumin (MAL)
Prealbumin (transthyretin)
Albumin
β-Defensin
Glycosaminoglycans (mucopolysaccharides)
Apelin
Angiotensin-I-converting enzyme (ACE) inhibitors & competitive substrates:
    enkephalins
    bradykinin
    substance P
    casokinins (casein-derived ACE inhibitors)
    lactokinins (whey-derived ACE inhibitors)
Albutensin A
Cathelicidin peptides
Motilin
Growth Factors
    Insulin-like Growth Factor I (IGF-1)
    Insulin-like Growth Factor II (IGF-2)
    Insulin-like Growth Factor Binding Protein-3 (IGFBP-3)
    Transforming Growth Factor Alpha (TGF-α)
    Transforming Growth Factor Beta 1 (TGF-β1)
    Transforming Growth Factor Beta 2 (TGF-β2)
    Fibroblast Growth Factor (FGF)
    Epithelial/Epidermal Growth Factor (EGF)
    Betacellulin
    Colony-Stimulating Factor-1 (CSF-1)/Macrophage Colony Stimulating Factor (M-CSF)

Granulocyte Colony Stimulating Factor (G-CSF)
Platelet-Derived Growth Factor (PDGF)
Vascular Endothelial Growth Factor (VEGF)

Hormones

Erythropoietin (EPO)
Estrogens
Gonadotropin-releasing Hormone (GnRH)
Growth Hormone/Somatotropin
Insulin
Leptin
Luteinizing Hormone-releasing Hormone (LHRH)
Melatonin
Procalcitonin / Calcitonin
Progesterone
Prolactin
Relaxin
Somatostatin
Thyrotropin-releasing Hormone (TRH)

Enzymes

Alkaline phosphatase
Amylase
Carbonic anhydrase
Fructose-bisphosphate aldolase / Aldolase A
Glycosyl transferases
β-galactoside α-2,6-sialyltransferase
b-4-galactosyltransferase
Matrix metalloproteinases
Peroxidase
Superoxide dismutase
Telomerase (?)
Thiamine pyrophosphatase
Uridine diphosphate N-acetylglucosamine (UDP-
    GlcNAc)
Xanthine Oxidase

Phospholipids & Milk Fat Lipids
    Phosphatidylserine
    Phosphatidylcholine (lecithin)
    Phosphatidylinositol (inositol)
    Phosphatidylethanolamine (cephalin)
    Sphingomyelin
    Fatty Acids
    Linoleic acid
    Dihomo-gamma-linoleic acid
    Alpha-linoleic acid
    Eicosatrienoic acid
    Prosaposin
    Saposins A, B, C, D
    Tocopherols
    Cholesterol
Antioxidants
    Glutathione (GSH)
    Glutathione precursors (Cysteine, Glycine and
    Glutamic Acid)
    Uric Acid
Glycoconjugates
    Glycogen
    Retinoic Acid
    Orotic Acid
Miscellaneous Proteins
    Nucleosides
    cytidine
    uridine
    guanosine
    Nucleotides
    cytidine monophosphate (CMP)
    uridine monophosphate (UMP)
    adenosine monophosphate (AMP)
    guanosine monophosphate (GMP)
    Polyamines

Putrescine
Spermine
Spermidine
Amino Acids
  Essential Amino Acids
  Isoleucine
  Leucine
  Histidine
  Methionine
  Lysine
  Threonine
  Phenylalanine
  Valine
  Tryptophan
  Non-Essential Amino Acids
  Arginine
  Cystine
  Glutamic Acid
  Alanine
  Tyrosine
  Glycine
  Proline
  Aspartic Acid
  Serine
  Vitamins
  Vitamin B1 (thiamin)
  Vitamin B2
  Vitamin B6
  Vitamin B12
  Vitamin E
  Vitamin A
  Vitamin C
  Vitamin D3
  Folic Acid (folate)
  Pantothenic Acid

Beta-carotene

Minerals
Calcium
Chromium
Copper
Iron
Magnesium
Phosphorus
Potassium
Selenium
Sodium
Sulfur
Zinc
Probiotics
Lactobacillus acidophilus
Lactobacillus bifidus (Bifidobacterium)

Appendix B:
Enjoying Powdered Bovine Colostrum

Colostrum is an acquired taste. Depending on palate and overall food preferences/experiences, some people do not like the taste. Also, every batch of colostrum comes from different cows, hence the variation in taste, smell, density and solubility. If you find the taste of colostrum objectionable, here are a few things you can do to make it more pleasing to your palate:

1) Combine Colostrum-LD® with room temperature water in shaker bottle; shake thoroughly; add a few ice cubes or let chill in the refrigerator before drinking.

2) Brew chai or matcha green tea and allow to cool (or use instant green tea powder); combine tea and Colostrum-LD® in shaker bottle; shake thoroughly; add a few ice cubes or let chill in the refrigerator before drinking.

3) Use one of these blender recipes:

Strawberry-Flavored
1 Tbsp. Colostrum-LD®
2 fresh/frozen strawberries (preferably organic)
4 oz. water
2 ice cubes, if desired

Blueberry-Flavored
1 Tbsp. Colostrum-LD®
6 fresh/frozen blueberries (preferably organic)
4 oz. water
2 ice cubes, if desired

Chocolate-Flavored
1 Tbsp. Colostrum-LD®
1 tsp. organic cocoa powder
Stevia (such as TruStevia), to taste
4 oz. water
2 ice cubes, if desired

Remember: For maximum effectiveness, do not combine Colostrum-LD® with a protein source (i.e., whey or other protein powder) or with any significant quantity of carbohydrates.

Appendix C:
Clinical Trials with Bovine Colostrum and/or Its Components

Study 1:

Title:	Gut Priming With Oral Bovine Colostrum for Pre term Neonates; Randomized Control Trial
Status:	Completed
Conditions:	Late Onset Neonatal Sepsis; I Necrotizing Entero colitis of Newborn; Feeding - Difficult, Newborn
Interventions:	Dietary Supplement: Bovine colostrum
Locations:	Egypt
URL:	https://ClinicalTrials.gov/show/NCT03926390

Study 2:

Title:	Feeding Bovine Colostrum to Preterm Infants
Status:	Completed
Conditions:	Feeding Intolerance; Extrauterine Growth Retardation; Necrotizing Enterocolitis; Sepsis; Meningitis
Interventions:	Dietary Supplement: Bovine colostrum
Locations:	China, Denmark
URL:	https://ClinicalTrials.gov/show/NCT02054091

Study 3:

Title:	Bovine Colostrum for Preterm Newborns
Status:	Recruiting
Conditions:	Enteral Feeding Intolerance; Necrotizing Entero colitis; Late-Onset Neonatal Sepsis
Interventions:	Dietary Supplement: Bovine Colostrum; Dietary Supplement: Preterm Formula
Locations:	China
URL:	https://ClinicalTrials.gov/show/NCT03085277

Study 4:

Title:	Bovine Colostrum as a Human Milk Fortifier for Preterm Infants
Status:	Recruiting
Conditions:	Feeding Intolerance; Necrotizing Enterocolitis; Postnatal Growth; Late-Onset Neonatal Sepsis
Interventions:	Dietary Supplement: Bovine Colostrum; Dietary Supplement: FM85
Locations:	China
URL:	https://ClinicalTrials.gov/show/NCT03822104

Study 5:

Title:	The Effect of 8-weeks of Bovine Colostrum and Soy Protein Supplementation in Rugby Players
Status:	Completed
Conditions:	Exercise Performance; Body Composition
Interventions:	Dietary Supplement: Bovine Colostrum; Dietary Supplement: Soy
Locations:	Canada
URL:	https://ClinicalTrials.gov/show/NCT02951923

Study 6:

Title:	Visnadine, Prenylflavonoids and Bovine Colostrum to Treat Vulvovaginal Atrophy in Post menopausal Women
Status:	Completed
Conditions:	Vulvovaginal Atrophy; Menopause
Interventions:	Drug: Visnadine, prenylflavonoids and bovine colostrum
Locations:	Italy
URL:	https://ClinicalTrials.gov/show/NCT03281655

Study 7:

Title:	Comparison of Bovine Colostrum Versus Placebo in Treatment of Severe Alcoholic Hepatitis: A Randomized Double Blind Controlled Trial
Status:	Recruiting
Conditions:	Alcoholic Hepatitis
Interventions:	Drug: Bovine Colostrum; Drug: Placebo
Locations:	India
URL:	https://ClinicalTrials.gov/show/NCT02473341

Study 8:

Title:	Bovine Colostrum as a Fortifier Added to Human Milk for Preterm Infants
Status:	Recruiting
Conditions:	Growth; Necrotizing Enterocolitis; Late-Onset Sepsis; Feeding Intolerance
Interventions:	Dietary Supplement: Bovine Colostrum (BC) / intervention group; Dietary Supplement: FM85 / control group
Locations:	Denmark
URL:	https://ClinicalTrials.gov/show/NCT03537365

Study 9:

Title:	Efficacy of Combination Therapy of Glucocorticoids and Bovine Colostrum in Treatment of Severe Alcoholic Hepatitis.
Status:	Completed
Conditions:	Severe Alcoholic Hepatitis in 'Extremis'- Defined by mDF>54
Interventions:	Dietary Supplement: Bovine colostrum; Dietary
Supplement:	Enteral Nutrition; Other: prednisolone
Locations:	India
URL:	https://ClinicalTrials.gov/show/NCT02265328

Study 10:

Title:	Effect of Bovine Colostrum on Toxicity and Inflammatory Responses
Status:	Completed
Conditions:	Acute Lymphoblastic Leukemia
Interventions:	Dietary Supplement: Bovine Colostrum; Dietary
Supplement:	placebo
Locations:	Denmark
URL:	https://ClinicalTrials.gov/show/NCT01766804

Study 11:

Title:	The Effect of Bovine Colostrum Supplementation in Older Adults
Status:	Completed
Conditions:	Sarcopenia; Osteoporosis
Interventions:	Dietary Supplement: Bovine colostrum; Dietary
Supplement:	Whey protein
Locations:	Canada
URL:	https://ClinicalTrials.gov/show/NCT01792297

Study 12:

Title:	Antiretroviral Therapy Intensification With Raltegravir or Addition of Hyper-immune Bovine Colostrum in HIV-1 Infected Patients With Suboptimal CD4+ T Cell Response
Status:	Completed
Conditions:	HIV Infections
Interventions:	Drug: Raltegravir; Drug: Hyper-immune Bovine Colostrum; Other: raltegravir placebo; Other: Hyper-immune Bovine Colostrum placebo; Drug: raltegravir and hyper-immune bovine colostrum
Locations:	Australia
URL:	https://ClinicalTrials.gov/show/NCT00772590

Study 13:

Title:	The Effect of Bovine Colostrum / Egg Supplementation in Young Malawian Children
Status:	Completed
Conditions:	Stunting; Environmental Enteric Dysfunction
Interventions:	Dietary Supplement: BC/egg; Dietary Supplement: Control;
Supplement:	multiple micronutrient
Locations:	Malawi
URL:	https://ClinicalTrials.gov/show/NCT03801317

Study 14:

Title:	Bovine Colostrum for Patients With Non Alcoholic Fatty Liver Disease
Status:	Completed
Conditions:	Nonalcoholic Steatohepatitis; Fatty Liver Disease
Interventions:	Dietary Supplement: Bovine colostrum powder
Locations:	Israel
URL:	https://ClinicalTrials.gov/show/NCT01016418

Study 15:

Title:	The Effects of Bovine Colostrum in Bone Metabolism in Humans
Status:	Completed
Conditions:	Osteopenia; Osteoporosis
Interventions:	Dietary Supplement: Colostrum supplementation for bone loss
Locations:	Greece
URL:	https://ClinicalTrials.gov/show/NCT04040010

Study 16:

Title: Safety and Efficacy of IMM 124-E for Patients
                With Severe Alcoholic Hepatitis
Status: Completed
Conditions: Hepatitis, Alcoholic
Interventions: Drug: IMM 124-E (Hyperimmune Bovine
                Colostrum); Drug: Placebo (High protein milk
                powder)
Locations: United States
URL: https://ClinicalTrials.gov/show/NCT01968382

Study 17:

Title: Colostrum and Inflammation
Status: Completed
Conditions: Diabetes Mellitus
Interventions: Dietary Supplement: Bovine Colostrum
Locations: Wales, UK
URL: https://ClinicalTrials.gov/show/NCT04602039

Study 18:

Title: A Trial of Enteral Colostrum on Intestinal
                Permeability in Critically Ill Patients
Status: Completed
Conditions: Critical Illness
Interventions: Dietary Supplement: Colostrum; Dietary
                Supplement: Maltodextrin
Locations: Islamic Republic of Iran
URL: https://ClinicalTrials.gov/show/NCT03186716

Study 19:

Title: A Trial of Enteral Colostrum on Clinical Out comes in Critically Ill Patients

Status: Completed

Conditions: Critical Illness; Infection Complication; Multiple Organ Dysfunction Syndrome

Interventions: Dietary Supplement: Colostrum; Dietary Supplement: Maltodextrin

Locations: Islamic Republic of Iran

URL: https://ClinicalTrials.gov/show/NCT03019250

Study 20:

Title: Effect of Milk Oligosaccharides and Bifidobacteria on the Intestinal Microflora of Children With Autism

Status: Completed

Conditions: Autism

Interventions: Dietary Supplement: Synbiotic; Dietary Supplement: Prebiotic

Locations: United States

URL: https://ClinicalTrials.gov/show/NCT02086110

Study 21:

Title: PTM202 and Modulation of Host Resistance to Diarrheagenic E. Coli

Status: Completed

Conditions: Traveler's Diarrhea

Interventions: Biological: E. coli strain E1392-75-2A; Device: PTM202 [bovine colostrum + egg]

Locations: Netherlands

URL: https://ClinicalTrials.gov/show/NCT03301103

Study 22:

Title:	Using Travelan to Boost Immune Response in Vitro to COVID-19
Status:	Active, not recruiting
Conditions:	Covid19
Interventions:	Other: Travelan OTC [hyperimmune bovine colostrum]
Locations:	Israel
URL:	https://ClinicalTrials.gov/show/NCT04643561

Study 23:

Title:	Safety and Efficacy of Oral Colostrum Derived Anti Influenza Antibodies in Healthy Volunteers
Status:	Unknown status
Conditions:	Influenza
Interventions:	Dietary Supplement: colostrum enriched with anti flu antibodies
Locations:	Israel
URL:	https://ClinicalTrials.gov/show/NCT01026350

Study 24:

Title:	Anti-LPS Antibody Treatment for Pediatric NAFLD
Status:	Completed
Conditions:	Nonalcoholic Fatty Liver Disease (NAFLD)
Interventions:	Biological: IMM-124E [a bovine colostrum enriched with anti-LPS antibodies]; Other: Placebo
Locations:	United States
URL:	https://ClinicalTrials.gov/show/NCT03042767

Study 25:

Title:	Therapeutic Approaches to Malnutrition Enteropathy
Status:	Unknown status
Conditions:	Severe Acute Malnutrition
Interventions:	Dietary Supplement: Colostrum high protein powder (Neovite); Drug: N-Acetyl Glucosamine (GlnNAC); Drug: Teduglutide; Drug: Budesonide
Locations:	Zambia, Zimbabwe
URL:	https://ClinicalTrials.gov/show/NCT03716115

Study 26:

Title:	Study the Result of Ayurvedic SUVED & Reimmugen (Colostrum) Treatment on Vascular Disease, CAD, CVA, DVT.
Status:	Completed
Conditions:	Coronary Artery Disease; Cerebro Vascular Disease; Ischemic Heart Disease; Deep Vein Thrombosis; Peripheral Arterial Diseases; Vascular Disease
Interventions:	Drug: SUVED; Combination Product: REIMMUGEN;
Other:	Grain flour placebo
Locations:	India
URL:	https://ClinicalTrials.gov/show/NCT02920125

Study 27:

Title:	Study Evaluating the Digestibility of Serum-Derived Bovine Immunoglobulin Protein Isolate in Healthy Adults
Status:	Completed
Conditions:	Healthy
Interventions:	Other: Serum-derived bovine immunoglobulin protein isolate (SBI); Other: Matching Placebo
Locations:	United States
URL:	https://ClinicalTrials.gov/show/NCT02017405

Study 28:

Title:	Effect of Lactoferrin on Polio Seroconversion
Status:	Recruiting
Conditions:	Poliomyelitis
Interventions:	Dietary Supplement: Bovine Lactoferrin; Other: Placebo Glucon D
Locations:	Pakistan
URL:	https://ClinicalTrials.gov/show/NCT04432935

Study 29:

Title:	Impact of SBI, a Medical Food, on Nutritional Status in Patients With HIV-associated Enteropathy
Status:	Completed
Conditions:	HIV-associated Enteropathy
Interventions:	Other: Serum-derived bovine immunoglobulin protein isolate (SBI); Other: Placebo
Locations:	United States
URL:	https://ClinicalTrials.gov/show/NCT01828593

References

[1] Centers for Disease Control and Prevention. Chronic diseases in America. https://www.cdc.gov/chronicdisease/resources/infographic/chronic-diseases.htm. September 24, 2020.

[2] Centers for Disease Control and Prevention. Radiation and your health. https://www.cdc.gov/nceh/radiation/nri/default.htm. January 7, 2014.

[3] Gofman, JW. Chapter 11: Ending of the Era of Radiation Therapy for Enlarged Thymus. https://ratical.org/radiation/CNR/PBC/chp11F.html.

[4] Heinerman, J. Fascinating colostrum: an ancient food for modern times. https://www.vibrantlifeinstitute.org/articles/heinerman.html.

[5] U.S. Department of Health and Human Services Public Health Service Food and Drug Administration. Grade "A" Pasteurized Milk Ordinance. https://agriculture.ny.gov/system/files/documents/2019/07/2017_PasteurizedMilkOrdinance.pdf.

[6] California food and agricultural code section 35602. https://law.onecle.com/california/food/35602.html. October 25, 2018.

[7] Milk & the magic of ISIS. *Isiopolis*, 2014 June 5. https://isiopolis.com/2013/01/26/milk-the-magic-of-isis.

[8] Centers for Disease Control and Prevention. Results: Breastfeeding rates. https://www.cdc.gov/breastfeeding/data/nis_data/results.html. August 26, 2020.

[9] Section on Breastfeeding. Breastfeeding and the use of human milk. *Pediatrics*. 2012;129(3):e827– e841.

[10] World Health Organization. Breastfeeding. https://www.who.int/health-topics/breastfeeding. November 11, 2019.

[11] Kuttner A, Ratner B. The importance of colostrum to the newborn infant. *Am J Dis Child*. 1923;25(6):413-434.

[12] Campbell B, Petersen WE. Antibodies in milk for protection against human disease. *Milchwissenschaft*. 1959;14:469-473.

[13] Fomon S. Infant feeding in the 20th century: formula and beikost. *J Nutr*. 2001;131(2):409S-20S.

[14] Sabin AB, Fieldsteel AH. Antipoliomyelitic activity of human and bovine colostrum and milk. *Pediatrics*. 1962;29:105-115.

[15] Liu Z, Li N, Neu J. Tight junctions, leaky intestines, and pediatric diseases. *Acta Paediatr*. 2005 Apr;94(4):386-93.

[16] White JF. Intestinal pathophysiology in autism. *Exp Biol Med (Maywood)*. 2003 Jun;228(6):639-49.

[17] Vaarala O. The gut immune system and type 1 diabetes. *Ann N Y Acad Sci*. 2002 Apr;958:39-46.

[18] Vaarala O. Is it dietary insulin? *Ann N Y Acad Sci*. 2006 Oct;1079:350-9.

[19] Oddy WH, Kendall GE, Li J, Jacoby P, Robinson M, de Klerk NH, Silburn SR, Zubrick SR, Landau LI, Stanley FJ. The long-term effects of breastfeeding on child and adolescent mental health: a pregnancy cohort study followed for 14 years. *J Pediatr*. 2010 Apr;156(4):568-74.

[20] Hayatbakhsh MR, O'Callaghan MJ, Bor W, Williams GM, Najman JM. Association of breastfeeding and adolescents' psychopathology: a large prospective study. *Breastfeed Med*. 2012 Dec;7(6):480-6.

[21] Horta BL, Loret de Mola C, Victora CG. Breastfeeding and intelligence: a systematic review and meta-analysis. *Acta Paediatr.* 2015 Dec;104(467):14-9.

[22] Jedrychowski W, Perera F, Jankowski J, Butscher M, Mroz E, Flak E, Kaim I, Lisowska-Miszczyk I, Skarupa A, Sowa A. Effect of exclusive breastfeeding on the development of children's cognitive function in the Krakow prospective birth cohort study. *Eur J Pediatr.* 2012 Jan;171(1):151-8.

[23] Strøm M, Mortensen EL, Kesmodel US, Halldorsson T, Olsen J, Olsen SF. Is breast feeding associated with offspring IQ at age 5? Findings from prospective cohort: Lifestyle During Pregnancy Study. *BMJ Open.* 2019 May 30;9(5):e023134.

[24] Victora CG, Horta BL, Loret de Mola C, Quevedo L, Pinheiro RT, Gigante DP, Gonçalves H, Barros FC. Association between breastfeeding and intelligence, educational attainment, and income at 30 years of age: a prospective birth cohort study from Brazil. *Lancet Glob Health.* 2015 Apr;3(4):e199-205.

[25] Centers for Disease Control and Prevention. Rotavirus Surveillance - Rotavirus in the US. https://www.cdc.gov/rotavirus/surveillance.html. November 7, 2019.

[26] Sarker SA, Casswall TH, Mahalanabis D, Alam NH, Albert MJ, Brüssow H, Fuchs GJ, Hammerström L. Successful treatment of rotavirus diarrhea in children with immunoglobulin from immunized bovine colostrum. *Pediatr Infect Dis J.* 1998;17(12):1149-54.

[27] Ylitalo S, Uhari M, Rasi S, Pudas J, Leppäluoto J. Rotaviral antibodies in the treatment of acute rotaviral gastroenteritis. *Acta Paediatr.* 1998;87(3):264-267.

[28] Mitra AK, Mahalanabis D, Ashraf H, Unicomb L, Eeckels R, Tzipori S. Hyperimmune cow colostrum reduces diarrhoea due

to rotavirus: a double-blind, controlled clinical trial. *Acta Paediatr.* 1995;84(9):996-1001.

[29] Davidson GP, Whyte PB, Daniels E, Franklin K, Nunan H, McCloud PI, Moore AG, Moore DJ. Passive immunisation of children with bovine colostrum containing antibodies to human rotavirus. *Lancet.* 1989;2(8665):709-12.

[30] Brüssow H, Hilpert H, Walther I, Sidoti J, Mietens C, Bachmann P. Bovine milk immunoglobulins for passive immunity to infantile rotavirus gastroenteritis. *J Clin Microbiol.* 1987;25(6): 982-986.

[31] Yolken RH, Losonsky GA, Vonderfecht S, Leister F, Wee SB. Antibody to human rotavirus in cow's milk. *N Engl J Med.* 1985;312(10):605-610.

[32] Huppertz HI, Rutkowski S, Busch DH, Eisebit R, Lissner R, Karch H. Bovine colostrum ameliorates diarrhea in infection with diarrheagenic Escherichia coli, shiga toxin-producing E. Coli, and E. coli expressing intimin and hemolysin. *J Pediatr Gastroenterol Nutr.* 1999;29(4):452-6.

[33] Shield J, Melville C, Novelli V, Anderson G, Scheimberg I, Gibb D, Milla P. Bovine colostrum immunoglobulin concentrate for cryptosporidiosis in AIDS. *Arch Dis Child.* 1993;69:451-453.

[34] Heaton P. Cryptosporidiosis and acute leukemia. *Arch Dis Child.* 1990 Jul;65(7):813-4.

[35] Derscheid RJ, Ackermann MR. The innate immune system of the perinatal lung and responses to respiratory syncytial virus infection. *Vet Pathol.* 2013;50(5):827-41.

[36] Li Y, Juhl SM, Ye X, Shen RL, Iyore EO, Dai Y, Sangild PT, Greisen GO. A Stepwise, Pilot Study of Bovine Colostrum to Supplement the First Enteral Feeding in Preterm Infants (Preco-

los): Study Protocol and Initial Results. *Front Pediatr.* 2017 Mar 3;5:42.

[37] Brunse A, Worsøe P, Pors SE, Skovgaard K, Sangild PT. Oral supplementation with bovine colostrum prevents septic shock and brain barrier disruption during bloodstream infection in preterm newborn pigs. *Shock.* 2019 Mar;51(3):337-347.

[38] Sun J, Li Y, Pan X, et al. Human Milk Fortification with Bovine Colostrum Is Superior to Formula-Based Fortifiers to Prevent Gut Dysfunction, Necrotizing Enterocolitis, and Systemic Infection in Preterm Pigs. *JPEN J Parenter Enteral Nutr.* 2019;43(2): 252-262.

[39] Juhl SM, Ye X, Zhou P, Li Y, Iyore EO, Zhang L, Jiang P, van Goudoever JB, Greisen G, Sangild PT. Bovine Colostrum for Preterm Infants in the First Days of Life: A Randomized Controlled Pilot Trial. *J Pediatr Gastroenterol Nutr.* 2018 Mar;66(3): 471-478.

[40] Ahnfeldt AM, Hyldig N, Li Y, et al. FortiColos - a multicentre study using bovine colostrum as a fortifier to human milk in very preterm infants: study protocol for a randomised controlled pilot trial. *Trials.* 2019;20(1):279.

[41] Pammi M, Abrams SA. Oral lactoferrin for the prevention of sepsis and necrotizing enterocolitis in preterm infants. *Cochrane Database Syst Rev.* 2011;(10):CD007137.

[42] Panahi Y, Falahi G, Falahpour M, Moharamzad Y, Khorasgani MR, Beiraghdar F, Naghizadeh MM. Bovine colostrum in the management of nonorganic failure to thrive: a randomized clinical trial. *J Pediatr Gastroenterol Nutr.* 2010;50(5):551-4.

[43]McConnell MA, Buchan G, Borissenko MV, Brooks HJL. A comparison of IgG and IgG1 activity in an early milk concentrate from non-immunised cows and a milk from hyperim-

munised animals. *Food Research International*. 2001;34:255-261.

[44] Hoban R. Distant Echoes of Slavery Affect Breast-feeding Attitudes of Black Women. North Carolina Health News. https://www.northcarolinahealthnews.org/2016/03/03/distant-echoes-of-slavery-affect-breastfeeding-attitudes-in-black-women. March 3, 2016.

[45] Black Breastfeeding Week. https://blackbreastfeedingweek.org. August 1, 2020.

[46] Centers for Disease Control and Prevention. When Breast-feeding or Feeding Expressed Milk is Not Recommended. https://www.cdc.gov/breastfeeding/breastfeeding-special-circumstances/contraindications-to-breastfeeding.html. December 14, 2019.

[47] Keim SA, Hogan JS, McNamara KA, Gudimetla V, Dillon CE, Kwiek JJ, Geraghty SR. Microbial Contamination of Human Milk Purchased Via the Internet. *Pediatrics*. 2013 Nov;132(5): e1227-35.

[48] Geraghty SR, McNamara KA, Dillon CE, Hogan JS, Kwiek JJ, Keim SA. Buying human milk via the internet: just a click away. *Breastfeed Med*. 2013;8(6):474-478.

[49] Miles, E. Why to Avoid Ultra-Pasteurized and Ultra-Filtered Dairy. Kalona SuperNatural [updated 2019 Aug 30] https://kalonasupernatural.com/why-to-avoid-ultra-pasteurized-and-ultra-filtered-dairy.

[50] U.S. Department of Health and Human Services Public Health Service Food and Drug Administration. Grade "A" Pasteurized Milk Ordinance. https://agriculture.ny.gov/system/files/documents/2019/07/2017_PasteurizedMilkOrdinance.pdf.

[50] Raw Milk Laws State-by-State. ProCon/Enclyclopaedia Bri-

tannica. https://milk.procon.org/raw-milk-laws-state-by-state. February 2, 2018.

[51] American Farm Bureau Federation. Fast Facts About Agriculture & Food - The Voice of Agriculture - American Farm Bureau Federation. https://www.fb.org/newsroom/fast-facts. Retrieved December 14, 2020.

[52] Kirshenbaum, S. Americans Are Confused About Food and Unsure Where to Turn for Answers, Survey Shows. The Conversation. https://theconversation.com/americans-are-confused-about-food-and-unsure-where-to-turn-for-answers-survey-shows-82124. August 24, 2017.

[53] Dewey C. The surprising number of American adults who think chocolate milk comes from brown cows. The Washington Post. https://www.washingtonpost.com/news/wonk/wp/2017/06/15/seven-percent-of-americans-think-chocolate-milk-comes-from-brown-cows-and-thats-not-even-the-scary-part. June 17, 2017.

[54] Centers for Disease Control and Prevention. Chronic diseases in America. https://www.cdc.gov/chronicdisease/resources/infographic/chronic-diseases.htm. September 24, 2020.

[55] Stelwagen K, Carpenter E, Haigh B, Hodgkinson A, Wheeler TT. Immune components of bovine colostrum and milk. *J Anim Sci.* 2009 Apr;87(13 Suppl):3-9.

[56] Wakabayashi H, Oda H, Yamauchi K, Abe F. Lactoferrin for prevention of common viral infections. *J Infect Chemother.* 2014;20(11):666-671.

[57] Silva EG, Rangel AH, Mürmam L, Bezerra MF, Oliveira JP. Bovine colostrum: benefits of its use in human food. *Food Sci Technol.* 2019;39(Suppl 2):355-362.

[58] Playford RJ, Weiser MJ. Bovine Colostrum: Its Constituents and Uses. *Nutrients*. 2021 Jan 18;13(1):265.

[59] National Institutes of Health – Office of Dietary Supplements. Dietary Supplement Health and Education Act of 1994. https://ods.od.nih.gov/About/DSHEA_Wording.aspx. Retrieved December 1, 2020.

[60] Ebina T, Sato A, Umezu K, et al. Prevention of rotavirus infection by oral administration of cow colostrum containing anti-humanrotavirus antibody. *Med Microbiol Immunol*. 1985;174(4):177-185.

[61] Ebina T, Ohta M, Kanamaru Y, Yamamoto-Osumi Y, Baba K. Passive immunizations of suckling mice and infants with bovine colostrum containing antibodies to human rotavirus. *J Med Virol*. 1992;38(2):117-123.

[62] Rump JA, Arndt R, Arnold A, et al. Treatment of diarrhoea in human immunodeficiency virus-infected patients with immunoglobulins from bovine colostrum. *Clin Investig*. 1992;70(7):588-594.

[63] Florén CH, Chinenye S, Elfstrand L, Hagman C, Ihse I. ColoPlus, a new product based on bovine colostrum, alleviates HIV-associated diarrhoea. *Scand J Gastroenterol*. 2006;41(6):682-686.

[64] Elfstrand L, Florén CH. Management of chronic diarrhea in HIV-infected patients: current treatment options, challenges and future directions. *HIV AIDS (Auckl)*. 2010;2:219-224.

[65] Kaducu FO, Okia SA, Upenytho G, Elfstrand L, Florén CH. Effect of bovine colostrum-based food supplement in the treatment of HIV-associated diarrhea in Northern Uganda: a randomized controlled trial. *Indian J Gastroenterol*. 2011;30(6):270-276.

[66] Playford RJ, Floyd DN, Macdonald CE, Calnan DP, Adenekan RO, Johnson W, Goodlad RA, Marchbank T. Bovine colostrum is a health food supplement which prevents NSAID induced gut damage. *Gut.* 1999;44(5):653-658.

[67] Playford RJ, MacDonald CE, Calnan DP, Floyd DN, Podas T, Johnson W, Wicks AC, Bashir O, Marchbank T. Co-administration of the health food supplement, bovine colostrum, reduces the acute non-steroidal anti-inflammatory drug-induced increase in intestinal permeability. *Clin Sci (Lond).* 2001;100(6):627-633.

[68] Kuipers H, et al. Effects of oral bovine colostrum supplementation on serum insulin-like growth factor-I levels. *Nutrition.* 2002;18(7-8):165-172.

[69] Leppäluoto A, et al. Bovine colostrum supplementation enhances physical performance on maximal exercise tests. *2000 Pre-Olympic Congress Sports Medicine and Physical Education, International Congress on Sport Science, Brisbane, Australia.*

[70] Buckley JD, et al. Bovine colostrum supplementation during training increases vertical jump performance. *2000 Pre-Olympic Congress, Sports Medicine and Physical Education, International Congress on Sport Science, Brisbane, Australia.*

[71] Davison G, Jones AW, Marchbank T, Playford RJ. Oral bovine colostrum supplementation does not increase circulating insulin-like growth factor-1 concentration in healthy adults: results from short- and long-term administration studies. *Eur J Nutr.* 2020;59(4):1473-1479.

[72] Marchbank T, Davison G, Oakes JR, Ghatei MA, Patterson M, Moyer MP, Playford, RJ. The nutriceutical bovine colostrum truncates the increase in gut permeability caused by heavy exercise in athletes. *Am J Physiol Gastrointest Liver Physiol.* 2011;300 (3):G477-G484.

[73] Davison G, Marchbank T, March DS, Thatcher R, Playford RJ. Zinc carnosine works with bovine colostrum in truncating heavy exercise-induced increase in gut permeability in healthy volunteers. *Am J Clin Nutr.* 2016;104(2):526-536.

[74] Keech A, Nwabuko U, Chikezie C, Wogu GUE. Peptide immunotherapy: a new direction in HIV/AIDS treatment. Advanced Protein Systems, Unpublished Research. February 2008.

[75] Wikipedia. Leaky Gut Syndrome. https://en.wikipedia.org/wiki/Leaky_gut_syndrome#cite_note-BischoffBarbara2014-2. Retrieved December 12, 2020.

[76] Wikipedia. Intestinal Permeability. http://en.wikipedia.org/wiki/Intestinal_permeability#cite_note-leakygut2012-3. Retrieved December 12, 2020.

[77] Katz KD, Hollander D. Intestinal mucosal permeability and rheumatological diseases. *Baillieres Clin Rheumatol.* 1989;3(2):271-284.

[78] Fasano A. Intestinal permeability and its regulation by zonulin: diagnostic and therapeutic implications. *Clin Gastroenterol Hepatol.* 2012;10(10):1096-1100.

[79] Centers for Disease Control and Prevention. Sepsis – Clinical Information. http://www.cdc.gov/sepsis/datareports/index.html. December 7, 2020.

[80] Fasano A. Intestinal permeability and its regulation by zonulin: diagnostic and therapeutic implications. *Clin Gastroenterol Hepatol.* 2012;10(10):1096-1100.

[81] Sturgeon C, Fasano A. Zonulin, a regulator of epithelial and endothelial barrier functions, and its involvement in chronic inflammatory diseases. *Tissue Barriers.* 2016;4(4):e1251384.

[82] Hałasa M, Maciejewska D, Baśkiewicz-Hałasa M, Machaliński B, Safranow K, Stachowska E. Oral Supplementation with Bovine Colostrum Decreases Intestinal Permeability and Stool Concentrations of Zonulin in Athletes. *Nutrients*. 2017;9(4):370.

[83] Eslamian G, Ardehali SH, Baghestani AR, Vahdat Shariatpanahi Z. Effects of early enteral bovine colostrum supplementation on intestinal permeability in critically ill patients: A randomized, double-blind, placebo-controlled study. *Nutrition*. 2019 Apr;60:106-111.

[84] Kleisiaris CF, Sfakianakis C, Papathanasiou IV. Health care practices in ancient Greece: The Hippocratic ideal. *J Med Ethics Hist Med*. 2014 Mar 15;7:6.

[85] Tramèr MR, Moore RA, Reynolds DJ, McQuay HJ. Quantitative estimation of rare adverse events which follow a biological progression: a new model applied to chronic NSAID use. *Pain*. 2000;85(1-2):169-182.

[86] Bjarnason I, Takeuchi K. Intestinal permeability in the pathogenesis of NSAID-induced enteropathy. *J Gastroenterol. 2009;44 Suppl* 19:23-29.

[87] Frenk SM, Gu Q, Bohm MK. Prevalence of prescription opioid analgesic use among adults: United States, 2013 – 2016. *NCHS Health E-Stat*. 2019.

[88] Peery AF, Dellon ES, Lund J, et al. Burden of gastrointestinal disease in the United States: 2012 update. *Gastroenterology*. 2012;143(5):1179-1187.e3.

[88] Peery AF, Crockett SD, Murphy CC, et al. Burden and Cost of Gastrointestinal, Liver, and Pancreatic Diseases in the United States: Update 2018 [published correction appears in Gastroenterology. 2019 May;156(6):1936]. *Gastroenterology*. 2019;156(1):254-272.e11.

[90] Centers for Disease Control and Prevention. Antibiotic-resistant Germs: New Threats. https://www.cdc.gov/drugresistance/biggest-threats.html?CDC_AA_refVal=https%3A%2F%2Fwww.cdc.gov%2Fdrugresistance%2Fbiggest_threats.html. October 28, 2020.

[91] Magill SS, O'Leary E, Janelle SJ, et al. Changes in Prevalence of Health Care-Associated Infections in U.S. Hospitals. *N Engl J Med*. 2018;379(18):1732-1744.

[92] Urology Care Foundation. Urinary Tract Infection (UTI): Symptoms, Diagnosis & Treatment. https://www.urology-health.org/urologic-conditions/urinary-tract-infections-in-adults#:~:text=A%20UTI%20is%20when%20bacteria%20gets%20into%20your,have%20at%20least%20one%20UTI%20during%20their%20lifetime. April 2019.

[93] Centers for Disease Control and Prevention. Antibiotic Resistance Threats in the United States 2013. https://www.cdc.gov/drugresistance/threat-report-2013/pdf/ar-threats-2013-508.pdf. Retrieved December 1, 2020.

[94] Casey JA, Curriero FC, Cosgrove SE, Nachman KE, Schwartz BS. High-density livestock operations, crop field application of manure, and risk of community-associated methicillin-resistant Staphylococcus aureus infection in Pennsylvania. *JAMA Intern Med*. 2013;173(21):1980-1990.

[95] Borissenko M. Malaysian TopGrow™ Piglet Trial. Unpublished Research. January 2003.

[96] Borissenko M. Malaysia Colostrum Piglet Clinical Trial. Unpublished Research. October 2004.

[97] U.S. Food and Drug Administration. Supporting Antimicrobial Stewardship in Veterinary Settings – Goals for Fiscal Years

2019 – 2023 – FDA Center for Veterinary Medicine. https://www.fda.gov/media/115776/download. Retrieved December 4, 2020.

[98] Kostich MS. Concentrations of prioritized pharmaceuticals in effluents from 50 large wastewater treatment plants in the US and implications for risk estimation. *Environmental Pollution.* 2014 Jan;184:354-9.

[99] Stephan W, Dichtelmüller H, Lissner R. Antibodies from colostrum in oral immunotherapy. *J Clin Chem Clin Biochem.* 1990;28(1):19-23.

[100] Kelly GS. Bovine colostrums: a review of clinical uses [published correction appears in *Altern Med Rev.* 2004 Mar;9(1):69]. Altern Med Rev. 2003;8(4):378-394.

[101] van Hooijdonk AC, Kussendrager KD, Steijns JM. In vivo antimicrobial and antiviral activity of components in bovine milk *and colostrum involved in non-specific defence. British Journal of Nutrition.* 2000;84 Suppl 1:S127-34.

[102] Ellison RT III, Giehl TJ. Killing of gram-negative bacteria by lactoferrin and lysozyme. *Journal of Clinical Investigation.* 1991;88(4):1080-1091.

[103] Playford RJ, Floyd DN, Macdonald CE, et al. Bovine colostrum is a health food supplement which prevents NSAID induced gut damage. *Gut.* 1999;44(5):653-658.

[104] Playford RJ, MacDonald CE, Calnan DP, et al. Co-administration of the health food supplement, bovine colostrum, reduces the acute non-steroidal anti-inflammatory drug-induced increase in intestinal permeability. *Clin Sci (Lond).* 2001;100(6):627-633.

[105] Kim JW, Jeon WK, Yun JW, et al. Protective effects of bovine

colostrum on non-steroidal anti-inflammatory drug induced intestinal damage in rats. *Asia Pac J Clin Nutr.* 2005;14(1):103-107.

[106] Cairangzhuoma, Yamamoto M, Muranishi H, et al. Skimmed, sterilized, and concentrated bovine late colostrum promotes both prevention and recovery from intestinal tissue damage in mice. *J Dairy Sci.* 2013;96(3):1347-1355.

[107] IARC Working Group on the Evaluation of Carcinogenic Risks to Humans. Some Organophosphate Insecticides and Herbicides. Lyon (FR): International Agency for Research on Cancer; 2017.

[108] Aitbali Y, Ba-M'hamed S, Elhidar N, Nafis A, Soraa N, Bennis M. Glyphosate based- herbicide exposure affects gut microbiota, anxiety and depression-like behaviors in mice. *Neurotoxicol Teratol.* 2018 May-Jun;67:44-49.

[109] Van Bruggen AHC, He MM, Shin K, Mai V, Jeong KC, Finckh MR, Morris JG Jr. Environmental and health effects of the herbicide glyphosate. *Sci Total Environ.* 2018 Mar;616-617:255-268.

[110] Muñoz JP, Bleak TC, Calaf GM. Glyphosate and the key characteristics of an endocrine disruptor: A review. *Chemosphere.* 2020 Oct 19:128619.

[111] Carr AC, Rosengrave PC, Bayer S, Chambers S, Mehrtens J, Shaw GM. Hypovitaminosis C and vitamin C deficiency in critically ill patients despite recommended enteral and parenteral intakes. *Crit Care.* 2017 Dec 11;21(1):300.

[112] Fleming S. US Life Expectancy is Falling – Here's Why. World Economic Forum https://www.weforum.org/agenda/2020/01/us-life-expectancy-decline. January 2, 2020.

[113] National Library of Medicine. Search Of: Bovine Colostrum Infants - List Results - ClinicalTrials.gov. https://clinicaltrials.gov/ct2/results?cond=&term=bovine+co-

lostrum+infants&cntry=&state=&city=&dist=. Retrieved December 1, 2020.

[114] Antonio J, Sanders MS, Van Gammeren D. The effects of bovine colostrum supplementation on body composition and exercise performance in active men and women. *Nutrition.* 2001;17(3):243-247.

[115] Centers for Disease Control and Prevention. COVID Data Tracker. https://covid.cdc.gov/covid-data-tracker/#data-tracker-home. Retrieved June 22, 2020.

[116] Cesarone MR, Belcaro G, Di Renzo A, et al. Prevention of influenza episodes with colostrum compared with vaccination in healthy and high-risk cardiovascular subjects: the epidemiologic study in San Valentino. *Clin Appl Thromb Hemost.* 2007;13(2):130-136.

[117] Belcaro G, Cesarone MR, Cornelli U, et al. Prevention of flu episodes with colostrum and Bifivir compared with vaccination: an epidemiological, registry study. *Panminerva Med.* 2010;52(4):269-275.

[118] Wong EB, Mallet JF, Duarte J, Matar C, Ritz BW. Bovine colostrum enhances natural killer cell activity and immune response in a mouse model of influenza infection and mediates intestinal immunity through toll-like receptors 2 and 4. *Nutr Res.* 2014;34(4):318-325.

[119] Ulfman LH, Leusen JHW, Savelkoul HFJ, Warner JO, van Neerven RJJ. Effects of Bovine Immunoglobulins on Immune Function, Allergy, and Infection. *Front Nutr.* 2018;5:52.

[120] Jawhara S. Can Drinking Microfiltered Raw Immune Milk From Cows Immunized Against SARS-CoV-2 Provide Short-Term Protection Against COVID-19? *Front Immunol.* 2020 Jul 28;11:1888.

121 Sly LM, Braun P, Woodcock BG. COVID-19: Cytokine storm modulation/blockade with oral polyvalent immunoglobulins (PVIG, KMP01D): A potential and safe therapeutic agent (Primum nil nocere). *Int J Clin Pharmacol Ther.* 2020 Dec;58(12):678-686.

122 Woodcock BG. COVID-19 and the orphan biologic polyvalent immunoglobulin - "Let food be thy medication" (Hippocrates of Kos c. 460 - c. 370 BC). *Int J Clin Pharmacol Ther.* 2020 Dec;58(12):675-677.

123 Sly LM, Braun P, Woodcock BG. COVID-19: Cytokine storm modulation/blockade with oral polyvalent immunoglobulins (PVIG, KMP01D): A potential and safe therapeutic agent (Primum nil nocere). *Int J Clin Pharmacol Ther.* 2020 Dec;58(12):678-686.

124 Jawhara S. Can Drinking Microfiltered Raw Immune Milk From Cows Immunized Against SARS-CoV-2 Provide Short-Term Protection Against COVID-19? *Front Immunol.* 2020 Jul 28;11:1888.

125 Borissenko M. Malaysia Colostrum Piglet Clinical Trial. Unpublished Research. October 2004.

126 Kshirsagar AY, Vekariya MA, Gupta V, et al. A comparative study of colostrum dressing versus conventional dressing in deep wounds. J Clin Diagn Res. 2015;9(4):PC01-PC4.

127 Gałecki P, Talarowska M. Inflammatory theory of depression. *Psychiatr Pol.* 2018 Jun 30;52(3):437-447.

128 Troubat R, Barone P, Leman S, Desmidt T, Cressant A, Atanasova B, Brizard B, El Hage W, Surget A, Belzung C, Camus V. Neuroinflammation and depression: A review. *Eur J Neurosci.* 2021 Jan;53(1):151-171.

129 Giffard CJ, Seino MM, Markwell PJ, Bektash RM. Benefits of bovine colostrum on fecal quality in recently weaned puppies. *J*

Nutr. 2004 Aug;134(8 Suppl):2126S-2127S.

[130] Satyaraj E, Reynolds A, Pelker R, Labuda J, Zhang P, Sun P. Supplementation of diets with bovine colostrum influences immune function in dogs. *Br J Nutr.* 2013 Dec;110(12):2216-21.

[131] Rudman D. Growth hormone, body composition, and aging. *J Am Geriatr Soc.* 1985 Nov;33(11):800-7.

[132] Rudman D, Feller AG, Nagraj HS, Gergans GA, Lalitha PY, Goldberg AF, Schlenker RA, Cohn L, Rudman IW, Mattson DE. Effects of human growth hormone in men over 60 years old. *N Engl J Med.* 1990 Jul 5;323(1):1-6.

[133] Cohn L, Feller AG, Draper MW, Rudman IW, Rudman D. Carpal tunnel syndrome and gynaecomastia during growth hormone treatment of elderly men with low circulating IGF-I concentrations. *Clin Endocrinol (Oxf).* 1993 Oct;39(4):417-25.

[134] Liu H, Bravata DM, Olkin I, Nayak S, Roberts B, Garber AM, Hoffman AR. Systematic review: the safety and efficacy of growth hormone in the healthy elderly. *Ann Intern Med.* 2007 Jan 16;146(2):104-15.

[135] Papadakis MA, Grady D, Black D, Tierney MJ, Gooding GA, Schambelan M, Grunfeld C. Growth hormone replacement in healthy older men improves body composition but not functional ability. *Ann Intern Med.* 1996 Apr 15;124(8):708-16.

[136] Polkowska-Pruszyńska B, Gerkowicz A, Krasowska D. The gut microbiome alterations in allergic and inflammatory skin diseases - an update. *J Eur Acad Dermatol Venereol.* 2020 Mar;34(3):455-464.

[137] Salem I, Ramser A, Isham N, Ghannoum MA. The Gut Microbiome as a Major Regulator of the Gut-Skin Axis. *Front Microbiol.* 2018 Jul 10;9:1459.

[138] Ghevariya V, Singhal S, Anand S. The skin: a mirror to the gut. *Int J Colorectal Dis*. 2013 Jul;28(7):889-913.

[139] Prescott SL, Larcombe DL, Logan AC, West C, Burks W, Caraballo L, Levin M, Etten EV, Horwitz P, Kozyrskyj A, Campbell DE. The skin microbiome: impact of modern environments on skin ecology, barrier integrity, and systemic immune programming. *World Allergy Organ J*. 2017 Aug 22;10(1):29.

[140] Aubert G, Baerlocher GM, Vulto I, Poon SS, Lansdorp PM. Collapse of telomere homeostasis in hematopoietic cells caused by heterozygous mutations in telomerase genes. *PLoS Genet*. 2012;8(5):e1002696.

[141] Haycock PC, Heydon EE, Kaptoge S, Butterworth AS, Thompson A, Willeit P. Leucocyte telomere length and risk of cardiovascular disease: systematic review and meta-analysis. *BMJ*. 2014 Jul 8;349:g4227.

[142] Willeit P, Raschenberger J, Heydon EE, Tsimikas S, Haun M, Mayr A, Weger S, Witztum JL, Butterworth AS, Willeit J, Kronenberg F, Kiechl S. Leucocyte telomere length and risk of type 2 diabetes mellitus: new prospective cohort study and literature-based meta-analysis. *PLoS One*. 2014 Nov 12;9(11):e112483.

[143] Paul M. Telomere Changes Predict Cancer. Northwestern Now News. https://news.northwestern.edu/stories/2015/04/telomere-changes-predict-cancer. April 30, 2015.

[144] Drury SS, Theall K, Gleason MM, Smyke AT, De Vivo I, Wong JY, Fox NA, Zeanah CH, Nelson CA. Telomere length and early severe social deprivation: linking early adversity and cellular aging. *Mol Psychiatry*. 2012 Jul;17(7):719-27.

[145] Blackburn EH, Epel E. The telomere effect: The new science of living younger. London: Orion Spring; 2017.

[146] Jogi R, Tager MJ, Perez D, Tsapekos M. Bovine Colostrum, Telomeres, and Skin Aging. *J Drugs Dermatol*. 2021 May 1;20(5):538-545.

[147] Fabi S, Sundaram H. The potential of topical and injectable growth factors and cytokines for skin rejuvenation. *Facial Plast Surg*. 2014 Apr;30(2):157-71.

[148] Aldag C, Nogueira Teixeira D, Leventhal PS. Skin rejuvenation using cosmetic products containing growth factors, cytokines, and matrikines: a review of the literature. *Clin Cosmet Investig Dermatol*. 2016 Nov 9;9:411-419.

[149] Torre C, Jeusette I, Serra M, Brazis P, Puigdemont A. Bovine colostrum increases proliferation of canine skin fibroblasts. *J Nutr*. 2006 Jul;136(7 Suppl):2058S-2060S.

[150] Kshirsagar AY, Vekariya MA, Gupta V, et al. A comparative study of colostrum dressing versus conventional dressing in deep wounds. *J Clin Diagn Res*. 2015;9(4):PC01-PC4.

[151] Vailati S, Melloni E, Riscassi E, Behr Roussel D, Sardina M. Evaluation of the effects of a new intravaginal gel, containing purified bovine colostrum, on vaginal blood flow and vaginal atrophy in ovariectomized rat. *Sex Med*. 2013 Dec;1(2):35-43.

[152] Nappi RE, Cagnacci A, Becorpi AM, Nappi C, Paoletti AM, Busacca M, Martella S, Bellafronte M, Tredici Z, Di Carlo C, Corda V, Vignali M, Bagolan M, Sardina M. Monurelle Biogel® vaginal gel in the treatment of vaginal dryness in postmenopausal women. *Climacteric*. 2017 Oct;20(5):467-475.

[153] Schiavi MC, Di Tucci C, Colagiovanni V, Faiano P, Giannini A, D'Oria O, Prata G, Perniola G, Monti M, Zullo MA, Muzii L, Benedetti Panici P. A medical device containing purified bovine colostrum (Monurelle Biogel) in the treatment of vulvovaginal

atrophy in postmenopausal women: Retrospective analysis of urinary symptoms, sexual function, and quality of life. *Low Urin Tract Symptoms.* 2019 Apr;11(2):O11-O15.

[154] Park HW. Longevity, aging, and caloric restriction: Clive Maine McCay and the construction of a multidisciplinary research program. *Hist Stud Nat Sci.* 2010 Winter;40(1):79-124.

[155] Most J, Tosti V, Redman LM, Fontana L. Calorie restriction in humans: An update. *Ageing Res Rev.* 2017 Oct;39:36-45.

[156] Institute of Colostrum Research. Glutathione and Colostrum. http://www.colostrumresearch.org/research/study-papers/glutathione-and-colostrum. Retrieved December 4, 2020.

[157] Centers for Disease Control and Prevention. Chronic diseases in America. https://www.cdc.gov/chronicdisease/resources/infographic/chronic-diseases.htm. September 24, 2020.

[158] National Institutes of Health – U.S. National Library of Medicine. ClinicalTrials.gov.https://clinicaltrials.gov/ct2/results?cond=&term=bovine+colostrum&cntry=&state=&city=&dist=. December 4, 2020.